ASSIP – Attempted Suicide Short Intervention Program

T0315316

About the Authors

Konrad Michel, MD, is a clinical psychiatrist and psychotherapist who has developed a model of understanding suicidal behavior based on the theory of goal-directed action and narrative interviewing. He is the initiator of the Aeschi Working Group – an international group of clinicians and researchers dedicated to improving clinical suicide prevention by developing and promoting patient-oriented models of understanding suicidal behavior.

Anja Gysin-Maillart, PhD, is a clinical psychologist and psychotherapist at the outpatients department of the University Hospital of Psychiatry Bern, Switzerland. She is head of the special outpatient clinic for patients who attempted suicide (ASSIP) and is a researcher of the Clinical Research Division at the University Hospital of Bern with a special interest in clinical suicide prevention. Her main focus is on the investigation of therapy processes involved in reducing the risk of repeated suicidal behavior.

ASSIP – Attempted Suicide Short Intervention Program

A Manual for Clinicians

Konrad Michel and Anja Gysin-Maillart

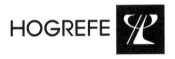

Library of Congress Cataloging in Publication information for the print version of this book is available via the Library of Congress Marc Database under the LC Control Number 2015938478

Library and Archives Canada Cataloguing in Publication

Gysin-Maillart, Anja
[Kurztherapie nach Suizidversuch. English]
        ASSIP--Attempted Suicide Short Intervention Program : a manual for clinicians / Konrad Michel and Anja Gysin-Maillart.

Translation of: Gysin-Maillart, Anja. Kurztherapie nach Suizidversuch.
Includes bibliographical references.
Issued in print and electronic formats.
ISBN 978-0-88937-476-8 (paperback).--ISBN 978-1-61676-476-0 (pdf).--ISBN 978-1-61334-476-7 (html)

        1. Suicidal behavior--Prevention--Handbooks, manuals, etc. 2. Suicidal behavior--Treatment--Handbooks, manuals, etc. 3. Crisis intervention (Mental health services)--Handbooks, manuals, etc.
I. Michel, Konrad, author II. Title. III. Title: Attempted Suicide Short Intervention Program. III. Title: Kurztherapie nach Suizidversuch. English

RC569.G9813 2015   616.85'8445   C2015-902740-3
                                                   C2015-902741-1

This present volume is an adaptation and translation of A. Gysin-Maillart & K. Michel, *Kurztherapie nach Suizidversuch: ASSIP* (2013, ISBN 978-3-456-85238-6), published under license from Verlag Hans Huber, Hogrefe AG, Bern, Switzerland. © 2013 by Verlag Hans Huber.

Translated and revised by Konrad Michel, Anja Gysin-Maillart, and Deborah Haessig, 2015.
The authors thank the Foundation Johanna Dürmüller-Bol for financial support for the translation.

© 2015 by Hogrefe Publishing

http://www.hogrefe.com

PUBLISHING OFFICES
USA: Hogrefe Publishing Corporation, 38 Chauncy Street, Suite 1002, Boston, MA 02111
                Phone (866) 823-4726, Fax (617) 354-6875; E-mail customerservice@hogrefe.com
EUROPE: Hogrefe Publishing GmbH, Merkelstr. 3, 37085 Göttingen, Germany
                Phone +49 551 99950-0, Fax +49 551 99950-111; E-mail publishing@hogrefe.com

SALES & DISTRIBUTION
USA: Hogrefe Publishing, Customer Services Department,
                30 Amberwood Parkway, Ashland, OH 44805
                Phone (800) 228-3749, Fax (419) 281-6883; E-mail customerservice@hogrefe.com
UK: Hogrefe Publishing, c/o Marston Book Services Ltd., 160 Eastern Ave.,
                Milton Park, Abingdon, OX14 4SB, UK
                Phone +44 1235 465577, Fax +44 1235 465556; E-mail direct.orders@marston.co.uk
EUROPE: Hogrefe Publishing, Merkelstr. 3, 37085 Göttingen, Germany
                Phone +49 551 99950-0, Fax +49 551 99950-111; E-mail publishing@hogrefe.com

OTHER OFFICES
CANADA: Hogrefe Publishing, 660 Eglinton Ave. East, Suite 119-514, Toronto, Ontario, M4G 2K2
SWITZERLAND: Hogrefe Publishing, Länggass-Strasse 76, CH-3000 Bern 9

Hogrefe Publishing
Incorporated and registered in the Commonwealth of Massachusetts, USA, and in Göttingen, Lower Saxony, Germany

Cover design: Daniel Kleimenhagen, Designer AGD

Printed and bound in the USA

ISBN 978-0-88937-476-8 (print) • ISBN 978-1-61676-476-0 (PDF) • ISBN 978-1-61334-476-7 (EPUB)

http://doi.org/10.1027/00476-000

Table of Contents

Preface

People with a history of suicidal behavior have their own individual stories, and so does this manual. The story started with the cooperation between me (K.M.), a psychiatrist who had undergone traditional medical training, and my friend Ladislav Valach, a qualified psychologist with a special interest in social psychology and, in particular, in what is called *action theory*. It was not until much later that I realized how much these two backgrounds in professional training differ in their "image of man" (*Menschenbild*), and how fruitful such an interdisciplinary collaboration could be.

Just as in the narratives of suicidal individuals, the story of this manual starts much earlier. It began during my training in the United Kingdom: On a morning when I arrived at the hospital and was told by the nurses that one of my patients, a 42-year-old woman with a husband and two preschool children, had just thrown herself under a truck. This experience had far-reaching consequences for me – not unusual for a young psychiatry resident. I started to read about clinical suicide prevention, and when I returned to Switzerland, I began a study of the clinical risk factors and the role of health professionals in dealing with suicidal patients. The question of what clinicians can do better to reduce the number of suicides has been an important part of my professional life ever since.

But let's return to my colleague, Ladislav Valach. During a coffee break, he made a provocative remark, which turned out to have long-term consequences: "Suicide and suicide attempts are not illnesses, but actions. You medical people have learned to understand conditions in terms of signs and symptoms – i.e., pathology – and make a diagnosis, but you have never learned to understand the nature of actions."

Despite my inner reluctance, I agreed to write a case description of a patient who, after a suicide attempt, had died by suicide 1 year later, from the perspective of action theory. The basic concept was that actions, including suicidal actions, are goal directed (e.g., to put an end to a state of mental pain), and that existential crises occur when a person is faced with a situation that is a threat to important life (or "life career") goals. In addition, action theory states that in everyday life, people use stories to explain and understand actions ("Well, this is a long story...."). As part of a study supported by the Swiss National Science Foundation, we tested the hypothesis that patients seen after a suicide attempt would feel better understood if the exploratory interview was conducted according to the concept of suicide as an action – as opposed to the traditional medical model, in which suicide is seen as a symptom of mental illness. In an action theoretical approach, the interviewer sees suicidal individuals as agents of their actions, capable of "knowing" the story behind a suicide attempt. We found that patients rated the therapeutic relationship as significantly better if the interviewer used a narrative approach (that is, opening the conversation by using the words *story* or *narrative*). This seemed to us an important insight, considering the serious communication problems between health professionals and suicidal individuals. One of the major problems in clinical suicide prevention is that patients who have attempted suicide do not comply with follow-up treatment. We hoped that with a narrative interview technique, a therapeutic relationship could be established early in treatment, which would be a starting point for an effective therapy. The key assumption was that feeling understood as an individual with one's own personal story would improve treatment motivation – one of the basic concepts underlying this manual.

To discuss the results of this qualitative study, we invited a handful of internationally recognized clinical suicide researchers to a conference in 2000. In a hotel in a mountain village of the Bernese Oberland called Aeschi, the group discussed fundamental problems in clinical suicide prevention, with the help of videotaped interviews. This experience generated so much enthusiasm that the group decided there and then to continue this type of conference and open up the discussion to others. There followed 10 years of Aeschi Conferences, which brought together some of the best clinical suicide researchers and therapists from all over the world. The so-called Aeschi Working Group published guidelines for dealing with people after a suicide attempt. In 2010 the American Psychological Association (APA), published the volume *Building a Therapeutic Alliance with the Suicidal Patient* (Michel & Jobes, 2011), which had emerged from the Aeschi philosophy. In 2013 the Aeschi conferences moved to the United States (Vail, Colorado).

During that time another fruitful collaboration was established at the Psychiatric Outpatients Department in Bern, namely with Anja Gysin-Maillart, with whom I coauthored this manual. Anja Gysin-Maillart familiarized herself with the technique of narrative interviews, and together we developed a specific brief therapy for people following a suicide attempt, which we called the Attempted Suicide Short Intervention Program (ASSIP). In recent years, we have treated well over 300 patients with this intervention program, refining, enhancing, and evaluating the therapeutic approach. It is thanks to Anja Gysin-Maillart's initiative that this manual has become a reality.

Konrad Michel
February 2015

Many years of clinical experience and scientific research form the basis of this manual. My (A. G.-M.) work has always been motivated by the view that patients need specific therapeutic steps following a suicide attempt, so that they become capable of seeing life as an option again. Over the years I was continually struck by the fact that this subject left not just me but also my colleagues baffled, if not helpless. Thanks to the prolific collaboration with Konrad Michel, my point of view started to change: Understanding suicide as an action and not a disease was a crucial factor. *Every patient has his/her own very personal and individual story, which needs to be understood.* I learned to understand suicide as a goal-oriented action with an inner logic, and I became increasingly fascinated by the collaborative process of developing, devising, and assembling the elements for a specific therapeutic intervention for people who attempted suicide. As my mentor, Konrad Michel gave me a thorough introduction to the field of suicide prevention. The regular Aeschi Conferences also played a key role. They provided an opportunity for professional and personal exchange of ideas with acknowledged experts, such as David Jobes, David Rudd, Marsha Linehan, Gregory Brown, and many others. In these very special small-scale meetings, I became familiar with concepts and models ranging from neurobiology to psychoanalysis and the latest developments in cognitive behavior therapy (CBT). The focus clearly was always on a patient-centered therapeutic approach.

The development of ASSIP took several years until we decided to start a first pilot phase to investigate its effectiveness. In this phase, the feedback from patients was of paramount importance. It was important to have our patients as experts with us, "on the team." It became increasingly clear that individuals who survive a suicide attempt need a safe place and hence a professional person, who will concentrate, along with them, fully and empathically on their individual inner experience. Therefore, we are thankful to our patients who helped us to better understand the suicidal process, and who continued to help us refine ASSIP and optimize it.

The time had come to start a scientific evaluation of the effectiveness of ASSIP. In collaboration with the Psychology Department of Bern University, we launched proper a randomized controlled trial with 60 patients each in the treatment and in the control group. As all of the patients were followed up over a 2-year period, the study took a long time to be completed. In September 2014 we got the final results, and these were very exciting, indeed. It seems that we had made a lucky choice with the therapeutic elements included in this brief therapy of 3–4 sessions, followed by regular letters over 24 months. The study gave me an opportunity to attend conferences and psychiatric institutions around the world and present our work. We were constantly met with calls for more information and to publish the therapy manual. Step by step, this ASSIP treatment manual came into existence.

With this manual I hope we have done justice to the patients' expert knowledge, and I express my heartfelt thanks for the invaluable contribution of every person who has participated in this project.

Anja Gysin-Maillart
February 2015

Acknowledgments

Our special thanks, first and foremost, go to all of the patients without whose willingness to take part in the study, it would not have been possible to evaluate this short intervention program.

We wish to thank all our colleagues who helped us develop, evaluate and implement ASSIP: Prof. Thomas Reisch, Prof. Hansjörg Znoj, Millie Megert, MA, Salome Bühler, MA, Pietro Ballinari, Dr. Leila Soravia, and Brigitta Feyer. We thank the crisis intervention team of the Bern University Psychiatric Services UPD, our colleagues, and the duty doctors for their cooperation and for referring their patients. Thanks also go to Prof. Thomas Müller, Prof. Franz Moggi, and Dr. Christoph Stucki, whose support made it possible to introduce ASSIP into our clinical work in the first place.

Our thanks go to Tino Heeg from Verlag Hans Huber, who wholeheartedly supported publication of the ASSIP manual from the very beginning. Our thanks also go to Robert Dimbleby of Hogrefe for his invaluable support of the publication of the English version of the manual.

My (A. G.-M.) warmest thanks go to my husband, Tobias Gysin, for his infinite patience and constant support of my work, but especially for editing the images in the treatment section of this manual. I thank my daughters, Sophie and Mia, for all of the magic moments we share, which help me time and time again to rediscover the inspiration I need for my work.

1 Introduction

Every year more than 800,000 people die by suicide, which equates to one death every 40 seconds (World Health Organization [WHO], 2014a). The number of attempted suicides is 10 to 20 times higher. After attempted suicide, the risk of a completed suicide is elevated 40 to over a 100 times compared with that in the general population (Harris & Barraclough, 1997; Hawton et al., 2003; Owens, Horrocks, & House, 2002). It is highest in the first 2 years (Suokas, Suominen, Isometsä, Ostamo, & Lönnqvist, 2001), and it increases with each subsequent suicide attempt and remains high for more than 20 years (Haw, Bergen, Casey, & Hawton, 2007; Jenkins, Hale, Papanastassiou, Crawford, & Tyrer, 2002). Therefore, special priority must be given to developing effective treatments for this patient group. In the 2014 research agenda of the Research Prioritization Task Force of the National Action Alliance for Suicide Prevention, the "Aspirational Goal Nr. 6: Ensure that people who have attempted suicide can get effective interventions to prevent further attempts" was given the highest priority of all goals (National Action Alliance for Suicide Prevention, 2014, p. 65). This is all the more important as so far there has been scant evidence that specific therapies following attempted suicide actually reduce the risk of a repeat suicide attempt or suicide over a long period. In clinical practice, all too often follow-up treatments – if they are offered to suicidal patients at all – do not even address the issue of suicidality at all.

In the prevention and treatment of suicidality, the main emphasis according to the traditional medical model has been on diagnosis and treatment of mental disorders – first and foremost depression. However, it is debatable how far this approach to the suicidal patient can actually affect suicide rates (De Leo, 2002). It has been argued that the mechanisms of suicidal behavior should be studied independently of any associated psychiatric disorder (Aleman & Denys, 2014; Linehan, 2008).

Various factors that hamper effective treatment of suicidality can be identified. One of these factors is that many patients do not comply with follow-up treatment. After a suicidal crisis, many individuals want to return to their normal daily lives as quickly as possible – that is, they try to forget the suicidal crisis as soon as possible. Up to 50% of attempters refuse outpatient treatment or drop out of follow-up therapy very quickly (Kessler, Berglund, Borges, Nock, & Wang, 2005; Kurz et al., 1988;). In a study, in which we interviewed patients 1 year after attempted suicide, the majority were unable to name a person they could have turned to for help, and a mere 10% said that they might have contacted a health professional. Most people in a suicidal crisis do not seem to think that this is a health problem for which one should see a medical professional. Too often people consider suicidal thoughts as something "private," which they want to keep to themselves, holding onto it as a possible escape in case they should find themselves in a situation with no other way out. Many individuals who have attempted suicide are ashamed and feel no one could understand them or their reasons. Many do not even understand their own suicidal behavior. Individuals at risk of suicide need a special way of communication and special opportunities to talk about their feelings, thoughts, and the background to their suicidal crises. Their motivation to engage in therapy depends to a large extent on the trust in the health professional providing therapy. What they need is nonjudgmental acceptance, empathic understanding, and a therapy model, which helps them to understand the mechanisms of a suicidal crisis, and to develop strategies for dealing with future critical moments in life.

In contrast to those who follow a traditional medical model, in which suicidal impulses are seen as an expression of a mental disorder, the authors of this book understand suicide primarily as a goal-directed action with its own inner logic. An action theoretical model provides a frame that gives room to the very personal experience of a person's suicidal crisis and its background. A key assumption is that people explain their actions with stories, and that the therapist must be open to listening without making rash attributions, because the suicidal person alone is the "expert" of his or her own story. In an action theoretical context, these stories explain how suicide can become a goal when important life and identity issues are threatened and no alternative coping or action strategies are available. In an acute mental state full of anguish, pain, despair, hopelessness, and helplessness, suicide may appear as the solution that will put an end to the unbearable mental condition.

Follow-up studies strongly suggest that when a person has attempted suicide, the risk of future suicidal behavior, including death by suicide, cannot be "cured." Once a person has tried to solve an emotional crisis with a suicide attempt, this behavioral pattern will quickly reemerge in similar future situations, not only because a suicide attempt provides a solution (albeit temporary), but also because very often it is associated with an immediate sense of relief. The prevailing view emerging from recent developments in suicide research is that, following attempted suicide, it is crucial to establish individual safety strategies with patients, for coping differently in future emotional crises (Stanley & Brown, 2012). For as many patients as possible to benefit, treatments targeting suicidality should be brief, focused, and, of course, effective (Chesin & Stanley, 2013).

Based on such principles, the two authors developed the Attempted Suicide Short Intervention Program (ASSIP), a brief therapy specifically designed for patients after attempted suicide. The key elements of ASSIP are:

- activation of the suicidal crisis by means of a video-recorded narrative interview in a safe environment;
- reactivation of, and distancing from, the suicidal mode through guided video playback of the narrative interview, identification of the suicide-specific emotions and cognitions, and development of new cognitive schemata, complemented by a psychoeducational handout;
- written formulation of long-term goals, individual warning signs, and safety strategies for future suicidal crises;
- video-prompted reexposure to the recent suicidal crisis, aimed at testing and strengthening the safety strategies;
- credit card-sized list of personal early warning signs and individual safety measures;
- continued contact with the patient for 2 years with regular correspondence.

ASSIP combines aspects of action theory, CBT, and attachment theory. A fundamental assumption is that an action theoretical approach to the suicidal patient will establish a therapeutic alliance in the sense of a "secure base" (Bowlby, 1980; Holmes, 2001), which will enhance the effect of the regular correspondence following the four treatment sessions. ASSIP is not a stand-alone therapy but should be offered to suicidal patients in addition to the usual clinical management and follow-up treatment.

2 Suicide and Attempted Suicide

2.1 Definitions

Suicide is the act of deliberately killing oneself. This definition includes intentional actions such as overdosing, hanging, shooting, etc,, and omission of life-saving measures – for example, refusing dialysis in renal failure. The concept of suicide as a "willed" action stands in contrast to the close association of suicide with psychiatric disorders (Barraclough, Bunch, Nelson, & Sainsbury, 1974; Isometsä et al., 1995) as well as the reports of suicide attempters who say that during the suicidal crisis they were in an out-of-the-ordinary state of mind, acting like in a trance (Orbach, 1994). The so-called rational suicide, where a suicide is believed to be a rational decision by a mentally healthy person is generally thought to be a rare exception, if it exists at all (Dörner, 1993).

Attempted suicide (Suizidversuch) was defined by Erwin Stengel (1964) as a form of deliberate self-harm limited to a short period of time where the suicidal person cannot know whether or not he or she will survive. Stengel referred to suicide attempts with only limited intention to die, as parasuicide or parasuicidal acts. Wilhelm Feuerlein (1971) sought a further differentiation based on the seriousness and the motives of the self-harm and introduced the terms *parasuicidal pause* (interruption of an unbearable situation) and *parasuicidal gesture*" (with a communicative or appellative aspect). The WHO/EURO multicenter study on suicide and attempted suicide (Platt et al., 1992) defined attempted suicide as

> an act with non-fatal outcome, in which an individual deliberately initiates a non-habitual behavior that, without intervention from others, will cause self-harm, or deliberately ingests a substance in excess of the prescribed or generally recognized therapeutic dosage, and which is aimed at realizing changes which the subject desired via the actual or expected physical consequences. (p. 99)

The WHO working group intended this working definition to cover the whole spectrum of life-threatening behaviors (WHO, 1986). Long-term self-harming behavior such as anorexia or substance abuse are excluded from the WHO definition.

Silverman et al. (2007) defined attempted suicide as a "self-inflicted, potentially injurious behavior with a nonfatal outcome for which there is evidence (either explicit or implicit) of intent to die." *Suicide attempt* is the term commonly used in German-speaking countries and in North America, while in the United Kingdom, the preferred terms are *self-harm, deliberate self-harm,* or *parasuicide,* terms encompassing all forms of nonfatal self-injury (Skegg, 2005). Attempted suicide usually includes episodes of self-injury with at least some intent to die; *self-harm* or *self-injury* are broad terms which range from habitual self-injury for emotional regulation without suicidal intent through to serious suicide attempts with high intent. Distinguishing between "seriousness of intent" and "assumed intent" is problematic (and not a distinction usually made in the German-speaking sphere). Intent is often characterized by ambivalence or even concealment. Often, the goal may be to initiate change, which can include finding release from an unbearable situation, finding a state of calm, ending overwhelming mental and emotional pain, and calling attention to one's suffering, as well as a desire to put an end to a life that has become unbearable (Bronisch & Wolfersdorf, 2012; Hjelmeland & Hawton, 2004). Most people who consider suicide as an option do not go on to make a suicide attempt. In a population-based study, only 7.4% of those with baseline suicidal ideation reported a suicide attempt over the subsequent 2 years (ten Have et al., 2009).

The term *attempted suicide,* as we use it in this book, includes self-harm with at least some intent to die but excludes habitual self-harm, which is typical in borderline personality disorders. *Suicidal behavior* encompasses suicide and attempted suicide. *Suicidality* here means ways of thinking and behaving such that someone accepts death as the possible outcome of an action (based on Manfred Wolfersdorf, 2000).

Internal and External Attributions

When we explain the behavior of others, we make attributions (ascribing causes and effects of actions). If we assume that the explanation for a behavior lies in the person himself or herself, we speak of internal attributions. If we assume that an external event is responsible for a certain behavior, it is an external attribution (Heider, 1958). As outsiders we usually only have fragmentary information to explain the behavior of others. This is especially true in the case of completed suicide, when we can no longer question the person. External attributions are based on theories and models we create to explain the behaviors of others. For example, media reports may explain the suicide of an adolescent with poor marks at school ("Poor marks at school: Suicide!"), thus not only badly simplifying the mechanisms leading to suicide, but also providing a simple and sensational model that may result in copycat suicides. The medical model, in particular, has a tendency to use external attributions, based on its tendency to search for the cause of pathology, and with its emphasis on mental disorders as the cause of suicide.

Buss (1978) argued that there is a fundamental difference between explanations by an outsider and explanations by the acting person. Outside observers tend to use causal ("why") explanations – for example, "Mr. B. took his life because he had lost his job." By contrast, the individuals concerned (people who have made a suicide attempt, or a suicide note left by the dead person) generally explain their action with a motive or intention: a "reason" as opposed to "cause" – for example, saying, "At that moment I saw suicide as the only possible way of putting an end to unbearable mental pain."

In suicide research, one way to find more person-centered explanatory models is by studying suicide notes (Leenaars, 1988) and through what is known as psychological autopsies (studies designed to do proxy-based diagnostic assessments). This method involves collecting all available information on the deceased via structured interviews of family members, relatives, or friends, as well as the attending health care personnel. In addition, information is collected from available health care and psychiatric records, other documents, and forensic examination.

2.2   Epidemiology

2.2.1   Suicide

It has been estimated that every year, around 900,000 lives are lost worldwide through suicide (Lopez, Mathers, Ezzati, Jamison, & Murray, 2006). Globally, suicide is the third most common cause of death in the 15–44 age group, and ranks second among 15- to 29-year-olds globally (WHO, 2014b). National suicide rates differ widely (see Figure 1). In 2011, suicide was the 10th leading cause of mortality in the United States, claiming more than 39,000 lives annually (McIntosh & Drapeau, 2014) and affecting many more, including family members, friends, neighbors, and colleagues. In the European Union, more than 58,000 people die by suicide every year (WHO, 2003). Despite increased prevention efforts, suicide rates are increasing (WHO, 2011a), and WHO estimates that in the year 2020, approximately 1.53 million people will die from suicide. The highest rates are found in Eastern Europe, in countries such as Estonia, Latvia, and Lithuania, and to a lesser extent, in Finland, Hungary, and the Russian Federation. There is a relatively consistent predominance of suicide rates of males over suicide rates in females, with an average of 3.6:1. The only exception is China, where rates in women are higher than in men, particularly in rural areas (Phillips, Li, & Zhang, 2002). There is a tendency for suicide rates to increase with age, predominantly for men.

In Switzerland, the death toll for suicide is about three times higher than for road accidents. The main suicide methods are hanging (30%), shooting (25%), and overdosing (14%). Males, who represent 75% of all suicides, tend to choose more lethal suicide methods. In international comparisons, Switzerland has a particularly high number of suicides by shooting, largely related to the widespread availability of firearms due to the militia army, which traditionally provided each member of the army with a personal weapon, kept in the household. Reisch, Steffen, Habenstein, and Tschacher (2013) showed that changing the practice in the Swiss Army of providing army members with guns to keep in the house had an effect on male suicide rates, and firearm suicide in particular. Generally, gun laws are an important factor influencing suicide rates (Miller, Azrael, Hepburn, Hemenway, & Lippmann, 2006). In the United States, 50% of suicides use firearms (McIntosh & Drapeau, 2014). A key element is the proportion of households owing firearms (Ajdacic-Gross et al., 2006). The introduction of new gun legislation in New Zealand, requiring control of access to and storage of firearms, resulted in a marked reduction of firearm-related suicides (Beautrais, Fergusson, & Horwood, 2006). Other preventive effects have been demonstrated for reducing packet size of analgesics (Hawton et al., 2001) or building barriers on jumping sites – so-called suicide hot spots (Beautrais, 2001; Reisch & Michel, 2005).

2.2.2   Attempted Suicide

Suicide attempts are estimated to occur up to 25 times more frequently than suicides (Goldsmith, Pellmar, Kleinman, & Bunney, 2002). In international comparisons, there

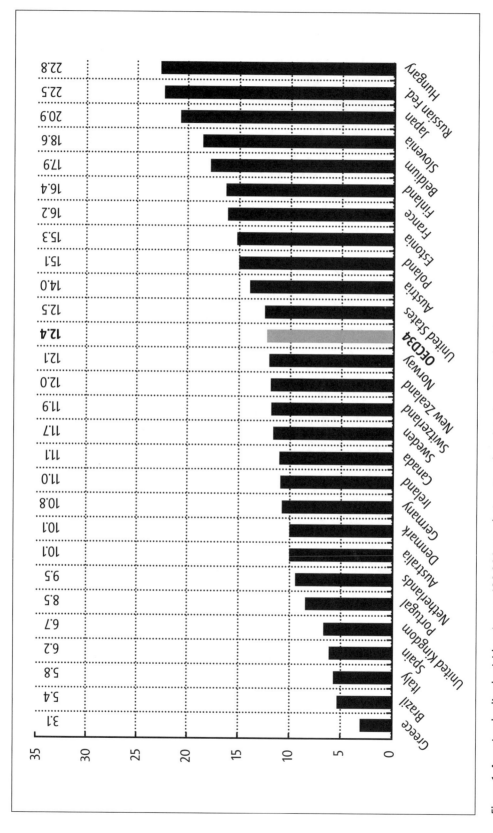

Figure 1. Age-standardized suicide rates per 100,000 population. Based on data from OECD (2013).

is a correlation between rates of attempted suicide and suicide (Hawton et al., 1998). Attempted suicide puts a heavy toll on health care resources. Emergency department visits and inpatient hospitalizations due to suicidal behavior are estimated to result in over 1 million hospital visits in the United States every year (Hoyert, Kung, & Smith, 2005). Surveys conducted in 2009 and 2010 indicated that an estimated 8.6 million US adults reported having serious thoughts of suicide in each of the prior years (Substance Abuse and Mental Health Services Administration, 2012). Nock et al. (2008), in a survey including 17 countries, found that the probability of attempting suicide was 29% in individuals with suicidal ideation, and 56% if they had made a suicide plan. Kessler, Borges, and Walters (1999) reported that, in the course of their lives, 72% of individuals with a suicide plan made an attempt.

In Switzerland, based on the data from Bern as a collaborating center in the WHO/ EURO Multicenter Study on Suicidal Behavior, a yearly incidence of 105.0/100,000 population was found (Reisch, Steffen, Maillart, & Michel, 2010), with a slightly higher percentage (57%) of women. The age group with the highest risk was 20 to 29 years. Forty-two percent had made previous attempts. The most frequent methods were overdosing, followed by cutting and jumping from a height.

2.2.3 Risk Factors and Protective Factors for Suicidal Behavior

Risk factors typically reflect a chronic but not necessarily imminent risk of a suicidal action. By contrast, *warnings signs* represent acute factors that imply immediate risk of suicidal behavior, and therefore require immediate intervention (Rudd et al., 2006). While there is a broad consensus that many suicide deaths are preventable, it remains difficult to predict and prevent suicidal behavior at an individual level.

Attempted suicide is associated with a high risk of mortality from suicide and other causes (Beautrais, 2004). It is the single most important risk factor for suicide (Harris & Barraclough, 1997; Hawton, Zahl, & Weatherall, 2003). The risk remains elevated for decades and is at its highest in the first year after a suicide attempt (Jenkins et al., 2002; Runeson, 2002; Suominen et al., 2004). Individuals who make suicide attempts also have high rates of reattempts. A systematic review found that an average of 16% of suicide attempters (range 12–25%) make a further attempt in the first subsequent year, with the risk being highest in the first 3 months (Schmidtke et al., 1996; Owens, Horrocks, & House, 2002). In the WHO/EURO multicenter study, 42% of males and 45% of females had made a previous suicide attempt (Schmidtke et al., 1996). Within 10 years, 28.1% of those who had been admitted because of a suicide attempt were readmitted for a further attempt, and 4.6% died by suicide (Gibb, Beautrais, & Fergusson, 2005). These findings indicate that those who are admitted to hospital following a suicide attempt are a group at high and enduring risk for further suicidal behavior and poor outcomes. They are an easily identifiable group of individuals who require short-term crisis interventions and longer term surveillance and management.

Psychiatric illness is a major risk factor – predominantly affective disorders, anxiety disorders, psychosis, and personality disorders (Beautrais, 2000; Harris & Barraclough, 1997). Affective disorders are present in 50–70% of suicides (Clayton, 1983). Between 25% and 50% of those with bipolar disorder make at least one suicide attempt (Goodwin

& Jamison, 1990), and their lifetime risk of suicide is 15% (Bostwick & Pankratz, 2000). In depression, patients may typically have negative cognitions about themselves and be subject to feelings of shame and guilt. They have a tendency to withdraw socially, and they have difficulties in confiding in others, which will increase the risk. Severe somatic illness increases the risk: Up to 50% of suicide attempts (especially in elderly people) have been associated with physical illness, often associated with chronic pain or physical disability (Stenager & Stenager, 2000).

Certain *demographic factors* are associated with increased suicide risk. Suicide rates are generally higher among males than females, but there are wide variations in the male to female ratio across countries. Attempted suicide is most frequent among adolescents and young adults (Armin Schmidtke, Sell, Wohner, Löhr, & Tatsek, 2005), while increasing age is a risk factor for completed suicide (Bertolote & Fleischmann, 2002). In the WHO/EURO multicenter study, being single, isolated, divorced, or widowed was associated with higher rates of attempted suicide. Other risk factors include unemployment and recent changes in the living situation.

Individual factors are related to a person's biography. Early traumatic experiences, such as sexual abuse, physical abuse, violence in the family, emotional neglect, loss, etc., are associated with suicidal behavior in adulthood (Bruffaerts et al., 2010). Stressful life experiences, such as divorce, separation, job loss, failing studies, etc., may act as triggers for suicidal behavior. The stress-diathesis model of suicide (Mann, Waternaux, Haas, & Malone, 1999) encompasses vulnerability factors such as psychiatric illness, familial and genetic components, adverse childhood experiences, and stress factors such as acute psychosocial crises – for example, experiences of loss, failure, and rejection. The concept of epigenetics has in recent years provided a bridge between biological and psychological vulnerability, related to early stressful experiences which can lead to long-term changes in the expression of genes related to the regulation of the hypothalamic-pituitary-adrenal (HPA) axis, and thus to a long-term dysfunctional stress system. Epigenetic factors are thus associated with reduced resilience[1] to stressful life events (Labonte & Turecki, 2010; Roy, Sarchiapone, & Carli, 2007). Furthermore, individuals with high impulsivity scores are more likely to act out on their suicidal impulses (Brent et al., 1994).

Media reporting on suicide can affect the frequency of suicidal behavior, due to an influence known as the Werther effect.[2] This phenomenon can be understood as a form of social learning (Bandura & Walters, 1963). Especially sensational media reports on the suicide of celebrities have been shown to lead to copycat suicides (Schmidtke & Schaller, 2000). Furthermore, sensational media coverage on suicide hotspots can increase suicidal behavior.

Protective factors have been identified. Being married or having children may be protective (Heikkinen, Isometsä, Marttunen, & Aro, 1995). Social skills, communication skills, self-confidence, the ability to seek help, or good coping strategies may be protective. Life-oriented perspectives, in private or work, are protective, as is an intact social network associated with high emotional and social support. Religious service attendance

---

[1] Defined as the ability to overcome crises by recourse to personal and socially mediated resources and to use this as a stimulus for development (Comer & Sartory, 1995).

[2] *Werther effect* is a term used in media research to describe the imitative effect that suicides by celebrities can have in a population. The term can be traced back to Goethe's novel *The Sorrows of Young Werther* dating from 1774, which is said to have launched a wave of copycat suicides.

is a protective factor (Kleiman & Liu, 2014; Stack, 1983). Regarding sociocultural factors, for instance belonging to the middle or upper social class, is related to lower rates of suicide and attempted suicide (Bronisch, 2008).

2.3   Models of Suicidal Behavior

Different models to explain suicidal behavior have been developed. Essentially, a distinction can be made among *medical, biological, sociocultural,* and *psychological models.* None of these can claim to be comprehensive.

2.3.1   The Medical Model

From the medical perspective, suicide and attempted suicide are a consequence of mental illness. This is substantiated by the findings of various retrospective studies into suicide, according to which 93% to 95% of suicide cases had symptoms fulfilling the criteria of a psychiatric diagnosis (Conwell et al., 1996; Harris & Barraclough, 1997; Robins, Murphy, Wilkinson, Gassner, & Kayes, 1959). Affective disorders have been found to be present in 50% to 70% of suicides, followed by substance abuse, personality disorders, and schizophrenia (Clayton, 1983). For attempted suicide, the picture is rather different. While the psychopathology in patients being admitted because of medically serious suicidal acts is largely similar to that in completed suicide, major depression appears to be less frequent in attempted suicide, especially in adolescents and young adults (Gibb et al., 2005; Michel, 1988). In the young, suicide attempts are often related to acute stress reactions – for example, those triggered by interpersonal problems.

Support of the medical model came from the so-called Gotland study (Rutz et al., 1989). In this study, general practitioners on the Swedish island of Gotland were given specific training in diagnosing and treating depression. In the following years, the suicide rate was significantly reduced, in contrast to rates on the Swedish mainland (see Section 2.6). Unfortunately, this study has never been replicated.

Clinical experience shows that too often symptoms of depression remain unrecognized (Freeling, Rao, Paykel, Sireling, & Burton, 1985), and consequently patients do not receive adequate (and life-saving) antidepressant treatment. Despite major efforts in training, the problem has remained largely unchanged, and several studies have confirmed earlier reports of alarmingly low rates of prescriptions for antidepressants among people committing suicide (Isacsson, Holmgren, Wasserman, & Bergman, 1994; Isometsä, Henriksson, Heikkinen, Aro, & Lonnqvist, 1994). One reason for the underdiagnosing of depression is that the signs of depression often are not obvious. Physical complaints may cover the typical symptoms of depression: Pain, autonomic symptoms, and gastrointestinal symptoms are common in depressed patients (Lin, Von Korff, & Wagner, 1989).

Typical Symptoms of Depression

- Persistent sadness or low mood
- Loss of pleasure
- Loss of interest
- Poor concentration or indecisiveness
- Low self-confidence
- Guilt or self-blame
- Social withdrawal
- Hopelessness
- Suicidal thoughts or acts
- Sleep disorders (early waking)
- Fatigue or low energy
- Loss of appetite; or (seldom) increased appetite
- Weight loss
- Loss of libido
- Psychomotor retardation or agitation
- Physical symptoms such as headaches or back pain, palpitations, gastrointestinal symptoms, difficulties with breathing

Depending on the intensity of the symptoms, depressive episodes are classified as mild, moderate, or severe. In a mild depressive episode, the patient usually feels unwell but, despite some loss of performance, is still able to carry out personal and professional responsibilities. In moderate depression, a person will have difficulties in coping with everyday demands at home and work, while in severe depression, the person will have serious functional impairment. A severe depressive episode may also be accompanied by psychotic symptoms, such as delusions of guilt or poverty, or hearing accusatory or defamatory voices.

Adapted from the *International Classification of Diseases* (10th revision, 2011b).

The traditional biomedical model is a causal one, which assumes that pathology is a result of a "fault in the system." In recent years, the role of depression as the main focus of suicide prevention has been questioned (Nock, Hwang, Sampson, & Kessler, 2010). Linehan (2008) argued that reducing symptoms of mental disorders is not sufficient to reduce the incidence of suicide attempts or suicides. Clinical experience shows that, although depression in particular and mental disorders in general are well-established risk factors for suicide, in the psychological treatment of suicidal individuals, it is not helpful to see suicide and attempted suicide as mere symptoms of a mental disorder.

2.3.2   The Biological Model

Exposure to early and repeated stressors may cause enduring alterations in the organism's physiology, cognition, and emotional response to the environment. The stress system has long been linked to depression and suicide – in particular, the functioning of the HPA axis, which regulates the stress hormones adrenaline and cortisol (see Figure 2). This system reacts to situations threatening homeostasis, with what is known as the fight-or-flight response (Cannon, 1929). For humans, trigger situations rarely involve external life-threatening dangers, but usually involve stressful psychological and psychosocial experiences, resulting in an increase of the cortisol-releasing hormone (CRH), which triggers the release of adrenocorticotropic hormone (ACTH) and which, in turn, stimulates the adrenal gland to produce cortisol. In the hippocampus, cortisol binds to glucocorticoid receptors, which normally, as a feedback mechanism, have an inhibiting effect on the HPA axis. This mechanism is disrupted in individuals with a dysfunctional stress system, leading to CRH hyperreactivity and a hyperactive HPA axis.

HPA axis function can be tested with the dexamethasone suppression test. Depressed patients whose cortisol level is not reduced after administration of dexamethasone have an increased suicide risk (Coryell & Schlesser, 2001). Early adverse life events resulting in a long-term hyperactive HPA axis have been associated with depression, anxiety disorders, and suicidality (Heim et al., 2009; Labonte & Turecki, 2010). A central element of the mechanisms involved in such epigenetics is long-term methylation, blocking the gene expression of the glucocorticoid receptor gene. This has been demonstrated, for instance, in a study with individuals who died by suicide and who had histories of early-life adversity (McGowan et al., 2009).

The stress system is functionally connected to the serotonin neurotransmitter system, which plays a central role in impulse inhibition. Numerous studies have shown an association between reduced serotonin availability in the brain and suicidal behavior (Arango, Underwood, Gubbi, & Mann, 1995; Asberg, 1997). This association appears to be inde-

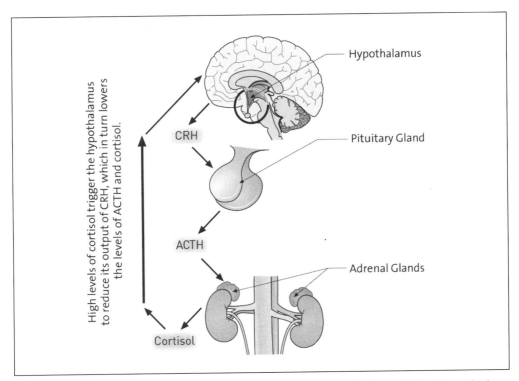

Figure 2. The hypothalamic-pituitary-adrenal (HPA) axis with its feedback regulation through glucocorticoid receptors in the brain. ACTH = adrenocorticotropic hormone; CRH = cortisol-releasing hormone.

pendent of the diagnosis of depression, although dysfunctional serotonin metabolism is also related to depression. Furthermore, the propensity to impulsivity and aggression is linked to suicidal behavior (Dumais et al., 2005) and a serotonin deficiency in the prefrontal cortex (PFC; Placidi et al., 2001). High levels of impulsive aggression and abnormalities in serotonin function are related to familial aggregation of suicidal behavior (Brent, Bridge, Johnson, & Connolly, 1996). Research has identified certain genetic factors related to suicidal behavior – for instance the tryptophan hydroxylase and the serotonin 5-HT2A receptor genes. Certain genetic variants of the serotonin transporter gene have been associated with depression and attempted suicide, depending on the number of stressful life events (Arango et al., 2001; Caspi et al., 2003). The influence of genes on suicide risk must be understood in the context of the interaction with life experiences (gene × environment interaction).

Decreased serotonin function associated with suicide is related to the function of the PFC (Oquendo et al., 2003). This part of the brain plays a key role in emotion regulation and cognitive processes related to problem solving and access to autobiographical memory, in conjunction with the hippocampus. Psychologically, impaired PFC function has been related to (1) a sensitivity to particular life events reflecting signals of defeat, based on attentional biases; (2) a sense of being trapped, related to impaired problem-solving capacities; and (3) the absence of rescue factors related to deficient life-oriented perspectives (Van Heeringen & Marusic, 2003; Williams & Pollock, 2001). Reduced problem-solving capacities in individuals with a history of suicidal behavior are a character trait – that is, these individuals perform significantly worse in psychological tests assessing executive functions, when compared with healthy individuals (Jollant et al., 2005; Williams, Mathews, & MacLeod, 1996). Switching of strategies as part of decision-making processes has been related to a network involving the anterior cingulate cortex (ACC) and the medial and lateral PFC (Carter, Botvinick, & Cohen, 1999; Paulus et al., 2001).

Seen in this context, suicide appears as "taking action but taking the wrong action" (Baumeister & Heatherton, 1996), related to impaired PFC function. The ACC and the PFC play a central role in self-monitoring and responding adaptively to stressors (Matthews, Spadoni, Knox, Strigo, & Simmons, 2012).

Consistent with findings from postmortem studies, a functional magnetic resonance imaging (fMRI) study on mental pain, in which patients were asked to recall the suicidal crisis, showed reduced neural activation in frontal cortical areas during the recall of the mental pain experience triggering suicidal behavior (Reisch, Seifritz, et al., 2010). The study also showed that, even when individuals are not suicidal, the suicidal state of mind – the suicidal mode – can be triggered by guided recall of the suicidal crisis. These findings suggest that the suicidal mode is stored in the neural circuitry, and is therefore a psychological mode as well as a neurobiological mode (see the Box "Suicidal Mode").

In therapy with patients who have made a suicide attempt, the neurobiological model may be helpful, not only because it can make the suicidal state (suicidal mode) more easily understandable for the patient, but also because it can reduce feelings of guilt and shame. Based on this experience, we have incorporated the biological model in our work with patients (see Appendix 3 "Suicide Is Not a Rational Act" and Section 3.6.3 "Ending the Third Session").

2.3.3   The Sociocultural Model

The French sociologist Emile Durkheim (1897) was the first to make a systematic collection of cause-of-death statistics from the 19th century in various European countries and to analyze the figures. He developed the theory that suicidal behavior is a consequence of the loss of social integration of the individual. Social integration has been found to play a role in the risk of suicide among immigrants (Wadsworth & Kubrin, 2007). Economic recession affects suicide rates (Platt & Hawton, 2000). Unemployment is associated with increased suicide rates, but the relationship is complex. Unemployment is often a consequence of mental disorders, a factor which itself is related to increased risk of suicide (Platt, 1984).

Cultural and social factors undoubtedly influence suicidal behavior. This is above all implied by the wide disparity in suicide rates and suicide methods found in different European countries. For instance, the high suicide rate in Hungary has been related to a "subculture of suicide" (Maris, Berman, & Silverman, 2000). The preference and availability of suicide methods can be seen as a cultural factor – for instance, the availability of firearms in a society (see Section 2.2.1) or the increase in suicide by charcoal burning in Asian countries (Chan, Yip, Au, & Lee, 2005). Similarly, media reporting on suicide has a strong cultural component (Pirkis & Nordentoft, 2011).

2.3.4   Psychological Models

Early models focused on *intrapsychic developments* preceding suicide. In the 1950s, Erwin Ringel (1953) examined 745 patients following attempted suicide, and on the basis of his assessments, he described the "presuicidal syndrome" with factors such as constriction, aggression reversal, and suicidal phantasies or flight into unreality. Pöldinger (1968) also focused on the development of a suicidal crisis, and described a process with a *contemplation stage* of varying length, an *ambivalent phase,* and a final *decision phase,* where the ability to distance oneself and to be in control is suspended. These models suggested that the contemplation of suicide does not usually lead directly to the realization of the suicide plan, but that there is an evolution over a longer period of time that can be influenced (intensified or halted) by many factors, and that suicidality is characterized by great ambivalence (Wolfersdorf, 2008). During the ambivalence of the decision-making phase, it is possible to intervene from a therapeutic point of view in many different ways to stop the suicidal development.

The Presuicidal Syndrome According to Erwin Ringel (1953)

To characterize the suicidal development, Erwin Ringel developed the concept of the presuicidal syndrome. In conversations with people following a suicide attempt, he discovered the following characteristics:

- Constriction with regard to thought (those affected see no alternative to suicide) and behavior (social withdrawal, isolation).
- Aggression reversal: Aggression is inhibited, with the aggression being directed at oneself.
- Suicidal phantasies: Flight from reality, thought contents are narrowly focused on suicide as the only way out.

The *interpersonal-psychological theory of suicide* (Joiner, 2005) states that certain preconditions are required for people to commit suicide. These are (1) the desire to die by suicide and (2) the ability to do so. The first condition will be fulfilled if two psychological states are present simultaneously over a certain length of time: perceived burdensomeness and a sense of low belongingness or social alienation, a mental state that will lead to a desire for death. The ability to die by suicide requires that the wish for self-preservation is to be overcome by a fearlessness of pain, injury, and death. This may follow repeated experiences of psychological pain in a person's life. Included in this model of suicide is the assumption that repeated suicidal crises and painful experiences will habituate individuals to pain and to the fear of self-harm. The implications of Joiner's theory for clinical suicide prevention lie in the clinician's attention to the levels of belonging and burdensomeness as perceived by patients.

Psychosocial developmental models interpret suicide in the light of a person's life story, where suicide emerges as a possible solution in times of crisis due to unsolvable difficulties, failures, or conflicts. Rich and colleagues (1991) found that the most frequent stressors were interpersonal conflicts, separation, and rejection, and less frequently, economic problems and medical illness. The frequencies of these stressors differed, depending on the life cycles in adult development. When questioned, most people who have attempted suicide say that in the past they had repeatedly thought of suicide as a possibility. It is in this context that Maris (1981) used the concept of a suicide career, or development toward suicide. This model stresses that repeated painful experiences lead to an increasing feeling of unhappiness, or clinical depression, both resulting in a more internalized interpretation of life difficulties and an increased suicide risk.

The influence of *environmental factors* on suicidal behavior is complex. Current models of suicide stress the interaction between genetic and environmental factors. A specific aspect of environmental factors is the exposure to models of suicidal behavior. Bandura's theory of observational learning (or modeling) is used to explain a wide variety of behaviors (Bandura & Walters, 1963). The modeling effect of suicidal behavior can be direct (suicidal behavior in the family or among peers) or indirect (suicide reporting in the media). Early exposure to suicidal behavior in the family and among friends is associated with an increase in suicidal behavior (Ventrice, Valach, Reisch, & Michel, 2010). The *Werther effect* refers to copycat suicides as the result of sensational media coverage (Phillips, 1974). For example, Sonneck et al. (1994) reported the contagious effect of media coverage of subway suicides in Vienna. Schmidtke and Häfner (1986) in their examination of the impact of the TV series *Death of a Student* demonstrated a considerable copycat effect. In clinical suicide prevention, in order to understand a person's background story of suicidal behavior, it may be important to ask about sources of learning about suicidal behavior.

Suicide in the *psychoanalytic model* is seen as an act resulting from largely unconscious mechanisms. The model is based on the theories of Sigmund Freud (1917), who, in his paper "Mourning and Melancholia," wrote about the evolution of suicidal behavior. In this paper Freud describes suicide in connection with depressive disorders. Due to a fear of loss, a depressed person is ambivalently attached to a loved and simultaneously hated object. The real, or imagined, loss of this object results in aggression that cannot be directed outward, and the ambivalently possessed object is internalized. Aggression is turned towards the *self* and manifests itself in self-hate and suicidal intentions. From a perspective of object relations, the inner conflict involves different internalized aspects of others, and the clinician should strive to understand the patient's suicidal dynamics (Bell,

2008). For many of these patients, neither separateness nor intimacy is possible. Malts-berger and Buie (1974) identified distinctive "suicide fantasies" – that is, unconscious relational dynamics leading to suicidal behavior. Suicidal phantasies are characterized by motives such as revenge and retaliation, but also a desire for symbiosis, devotion, and loy-alty. In the psychoanalytic concept of suicidality, the interaction of a triggering event with an internal conflict (experiences of separation and loss, conflict with partner, rejection) is key. Maltsberger (2004) argued that suicide is a traumatic state of disintegration, in which, for the person totally overwhelmed by overpowering emotions, the attack on the body has a calming effect. The impaired reality testing is understood as a transient psychotic moment. For the suicidal person, the break up of the self and its total disintegration are a possibility, which is a fear that is felt to be far worse than physical death.

Other psychoanalytic authors see a narcissistic crisis as the main reason for suicidal acts (Henseler, 1974). At the forefront of this theory is a disturbance in the narcissisticly unstable self-organization. Narcissistic individuals are vulnerable and strive to maintain and believe in a grandiose "false self" as a means of survival. One of the characteristics of suicide-vulnerable persons is their reliance on self-objects – that is, exterior sustaining resources to help moderate and regulate affect (Kohut, 1971). In an emotional crisis even the slightest insult is experienced as a "narcissistic catastrophe." The dominating feeling that follows is one of worthlessness and no longer being important to anyone.

Attachment theory has its origins in psychoanalysis as well as in evolutionary biol-ogy. The attachment style acquired in childhood plays an essential role for a person's capacity for emotional regulation (Bowlby, 1977). Mary Ainsworth and colleagues (Ain-sworth, 1989) distinguished among four types of attachment patterns: secure, ambivalent, avoidant, and disorganized attachment. People with a secure attachment style develop a positive working model of themselves and of social relationships. They have mental representations of others as being helpful while viewing themselves as worthy of respect, and generally tend to experience stable interpersonal relationships and emotional stabil-ity, which safeguard against suicide. Adults with avoidant, ambivalent, or disorganized attachment styles have a negative self-image and are at increased risk of emotional insta-bility, facilitating psychiatric disturbance and suicidal crises. Suicidal behavior will arise when arousal is at its height, and may be seen as a person's attempt to regulate unbearable affect.

A key finding in the attachment literature is the relationship between the security of attachment and the reflexive function, the capacity to talk cogently and coherently about oneself and one's difficulties. Thus, attachment theory provides a frame for storytell-ing, story listening, and story understanding to form the heart of psychotherapy sessions (Holmes, 2001). Suicide is the result of a collapse of an individual's attachment patterns. With no one to turn to when threatened, a person may become intensely vulnerable, "feel-ing alone in the midst of unbearable emotional states" (Allen, 2011). Death may be imag-ined as a preferable alternative to extreme emotional isolation.

On the basis of attachment theory, Fonagy et al. (2004) addressed the consequences of insecure and disorganized attachment styles in borderline personality disorders. People with a borderline personality disorder have a tendency to excessive stress reactions, and in this context, to self-harm and suicidal behavior. Bateman and Fonagy (2008) attribute this behavior to a lack of "mentalizing." *Mentalization* has been defined as the ability "to see oneself from the outside, and others from the inside" (Holmes, 2006). Mentalizing is understood as a developmental process emerging in the course of the first 5 years of life, and then elaborated throughout the psychological life cycle. Mentalization is impaired during stress reactions triggered by the inability to cope with – for instance, an impending separation – explaining the tendency toward impulsive and unreflective behavior. In this context, suicide is seen as a failure of mentalizing – that is, a failure of the capacity to differentiate thoughts and feelings from "reality" (Holmes, 2011).

A key element of attachment theory is the concept of the *secure base*. The secure base is a central element of Bowlby's concept of parenting as

> the provision by both parents of a secure base from which a child or an adolescent can make sorties into the outside world and to which he can return knowing for sure that he will be welcomed when he gets there, nourished physically and emotionally, comforted if distressed, reassured if frightened. (Bowlby, 1988, p. 11)

The Therapist as "Secure Base"

The concept of the secure base is a key element in attachment theory (Bowlby, 1988). *Secure base* originally referred to Bowlby's concept of parenting. This is characterized by being emotionally available; sensitive to the needs of the child; and ready to respond, encourage, assist when necessary, comfort when distressed, and reassure when frightened. The sensitivity of the caregiver is essential: The child needs security *and* autonomy. In providing the patient with a secure base from which to explore and express thoughts and feelings, the therapist's role is analogous to that of a mother who provides her child with a secure base from which to explore the world (Bowlby, 1988, p. 140). The concept of attachment in the secure base model differs fundamentally from that of dependence. Attachment security is characterized by sensitive and responsive caregiving. The attachment model of a responsive caregiver who is likely to promote secure attachment corresponds to that of a good therapist who is characterized as sensitive, responsive, consistent, reliable, and psychologically minded (Holmes, 2001, p. 16).

The concept of the secure base plays an essential part in the ASSIP brief therapy: The therapist's approach to the patient's suicidality, starting with a narrative interview, lays the ground for a therapeutic alliance in the collaborative exploration of the mechanisms leading to suicidal behavior. In the first two sessions, patients experience the painful emotions associated with their suicidal state, in the context of an attachment relationship, in which they are no longer alone but experience *their mind being held in mind by the therapist* (Allen, 2011). This experience, in turn, will help to enhance their capacity to mentalize in the midst of emotional states rather than being emotionally overwhelmed in a nonmentalizing and helpless suicidal state. Regarding the fact that after attempted suicide, the risk for future suicidal behavior is greatly increased, a long-term "secure anchorage" based on a secure base experience established during the face-to-face sessions is considered to be an important effect factor of ASSIP. The importance of the sense of a secure base (or anchorage) is illustrated by the following extract from a letter written by one of the ASSIP patients 1 year after the suicide attempt:

> *You will be surprised by my report, but unfortunately the situation in the past few weeks has still been very difficult for me.... The feelings of hopelessness led straight away to thoughts about suicide, which sometimes lasted for days. At this time the possibility of getting in touch with you was the only thing that helped me to believe that I could survive this situation unharmed. Since then things have returned to normal a little, so that I am much more stable at the moment.*

Attachment theory maintains that attachment behavior characterizes human behavior "from the cradle to the grave" (Bowlby, 1977a). When all goes well, attachment behavior is usually not apparent; it is seen mainly in moments when a person's inner equilibrium is threatened (according to John Bowlby: "in times of calamity"). Throughout life, we form new attachment relationships. These relationships serve the same function for adults as for children; they provide a secure base, which offers comfort and reassurance and, at the same time, allows us to operate in the world with confidence. When feeling threatened, proximity to a "secure base" person is sought for protection (see the Box "The Therapist as 'Secure Base'").

The *cognitive behavior model* of suicide starts from the presumption that the way people think about and interpret life events plays a causal role in their emotional and behavioral responses to those events (Beck, 1976). Consistency theory (Grawe, 2004) assumes that individuals have a strong need to seek harmony or compatibility between motivational goals and actual perceptions of reality. Congruence is understood as the harmony or compatibility between motivational goals and the actual perception of reality. Incongruence arises in an experience of a mismatch, or gap, between an actual experience (perception) and a goal. Suicide as a behavior emerges when an individual is in a state of strong incongruent signals. In this context, suicide is – although destructive – a way of reducing the unbearable tension caused by increasing incongruence. Baumeister (1990) described suicide as escape from a self that has become unbearable, with individuals blaming themselves for failures and disappointments in their life. The consequence is the cognitive collapse ("deconstruction") of one's self. In such moments, long-term perspectives do not exist, and life becomes meaningless. Negative cognitions about oneself, one's environment, and the future emerge (cognitive triad).

Suicide is seen as derived from specific dysfunctional cognitions – that is, individuals viewing their experiences and situations negatively, believing that attempts to solve the problems would end in failure. Stressors can be internal (negative thoughts, feelings, physical sensations) or external (interpersonal tension, rejection, loss). Suicidal individuals have a strong tendency to maintain negative perceptions of themselves, of the people around them, and of the future. The consequence is a feeling of hopelessness and the conviction that suicide is the only solution that can change this situation. Typical dysfunctional negative cognitions, as listed by Rudd, Joiner, and Rajab (2001, p. 29), include

- "My life is hopeless"
- "I don't deserve to live, I'm worthless"
- "I can't solve this"
- "Nothing's going to change"
- "I can't stand the pain anymore"

Dysfunctional cognitions evolve from schemas acquired throughout life and tend to be triggered automatically by specific events. Repeated emotional crises associated with suicidal behavior will lead to the creation of a *suicidal mode,* a cognitive-affective-behavioral reaction pattern (see Box "The Suicidal Mode").

The Suicidal Mode

The term *mode* was introduced by Beck (1996) and is used for acute mental states whose function is to prepare the organism to deal with exceptional and threatening situations. Modes encompass cognitions, emotions, physiological symptoms, and behavior patterns. The four systems work in synchrony when triggered either internally (e.g., by a thought, feeling, or image) or externally (situations, places, people, or things). In suicide research, the term *suicidal mode* has proven particularly useful in understanding sudden suicidal states, as reported by many patients (Rudd, 2000).

Emotionally, the acute state is usually experienced as mental pain, often accompanied by strong feelings of anger, anxiety, embarrassment, humiliation, and shame. Dissociative symptoms such as emotional numbing, detachment from body, and indifference to physical pain are frequent in the acute suicidal state of mind (Orbach, 1994).

Cognition is dominated by the suicidal belief system, characterized by pervasive hopelessness, with the individual seeing no other solution to put an end to an unbearable mental state (Rudd & Brown, 2011; Rudd et al., 2001). In an acute suicidal crisis, the focus on long-term life goals is lost.

Bodily functions are altered, reflecting an acute state of stress (arousal, accompanied by autonomic, motor, and sensory system activation).

The behavioral system is activated, often experienced as an impulse for flight. Included are suicide-related behaviors such as planning, preparing, and carrying out acts of self-harm.

A suicidal mode typically has an on/off mechanism and can occur suddenly – for some patients seemingly out of the blue. The suicidal mode is time-limited. One of the aims of therapy is to educate suicidal individuals so that they learn to recognize early warning signs and that they can use specific skills to cope with a mental pain experience, by engaging safety strategies. These skills should focus on typical trigger situations and emotion regulation.

The CBT model emphasizes the therapist's role as an active and engaged expert, with a focus on three areas: symptom management (crisis resolution), skill building, and personality development (Rudd et al., 2001, p. 43). Rudd and colleagues (2009) identified common elements of treatments that work, distilled from a review of available randomized clinical trials targeting suicidality. One such element is providing patients with *simple and understandable models for suicidality*. A clear and consistent therapeutic model is a strong factor in facilitating hope, with likely positive implications for motivation, commitment, and overall treatment engagement.

In terms of decision making, the *dual-processing theory* (Epstein, Pacini, Denes-Raj, & Heier, 1996; Stanovich & West, 2000) understands suicidal behavior as intuitive and automatic, typical for *System 1* processing. This system of decision making typically operates within an emotional context and has a tendency to jump to conclusions on the basis of very limited evidence. The theory implies that in suicidal individuals, the correctional mechanism of System 2, which involves cognitive control of behavior, does not stop the System 1 engaging in a suicidal action (Michel, 2014). In this model, suicide appears as "taking action but taking the wrong action" (Baumeister & Heatherton, 1996).

The *action theoretical model* focuses on the notion that goals and goal-directed behavior are central for the understanding of human behavior (Carver & Scheier, 1990). Action theory, or the theory of goal-directed action, represents a developmental systems theory to explain actions in terms of goals (Valach, Young, & Lynam, 2002). Actions are associated with cognitive and emotional processes, which involve planning, steering, monitoring, and decision making. These processes can be conscious or unconscious in nature. Actions are related to mid- and long-term goal-oriented systems, such as projects and life-career or identity goals. Actions are socially influenced and regulated (Valach, Michel, Young, & Dey, 2006). Translated into practical terms, this may mean the influence of friends, media, etc. on the individual, but also that of the therapist or the hospital staff.

Michel and Valach (1997) proposed a model of suicidal behavior based on action theory. In this model, suicide is seen as an alternative to original life-career goals, which may relate to relationship-related goals (to maintain a good marriage) or work-related goals (to achieve a secure income to support the family). In critical times, when a person's self-evaluation is negative ("I am a failure"), suicide may emerge as a possible solution to a subjectively unbearable situation. In these moments, suicide may temporarily become the main hierarchical goal, replacing life-oriented goals. An emotional reaction to a triggering event serves as an energizer, which may transform an intention into a final action (Valach, Young, & Michel, 2011). After a suicide attempt, life-oriented goals may soon reemerge. For example, it is not uncommon that after suicide attempt, a patient wants to go to work the next morning. A developmental systems theoretical model implies that the way people make sense of the actions of others' and the way people communicate their own actions are through narratives. With conscious representations of goal-directed processes being an integral aspect of intention building and goal setting, individuals are capable of giving their accounts of the processes which precede suicidal behavior, and are thus able to explain a suicide action (Valach, Michel, Young, & Dey, 2002). The patient's narrative is the basis of a therapeutic alliance (Michel & Valach, 2011). It is a subjective account, which reflects the patient's inner experience. Without the patient's story, therapy focusing on the patient's suicidality is constrained if not impossible.

2.4   Prevention of Suicidal Behavior

In the WHO Mental Health Action Plan 2013–2020 (WHO, 2013), WHO member states have committed themselves to working toward the global target of reducing the suicide rate in countries by 10% by 2020. Suicidal behavior is an extremely multifactorial mental health problem. It is therefore not surprising that a successful prevention project such as the Alliance Against Depression (Nürnberger Bündnis gegen Depression, http://www.buendnis-depression.de) used a whole range of different approaches (Hegerl, Althaus, Schmidtke, & Niklewski, 2006). These included public relations activities; educating the general public about depression and its treatment; directives for media coverage; cooperation with multipliers such as church ministers, teachers, police, nurses, etc.; cooperation with general practitioners (GPs); support for patients and their families. In the campaign's second year, a impressive reduction of 26%, and in the third year a reduction of 36%, in the number of suicide attempts was recorded. Elements of the Nürnberg study were subsequently adopted by programs of the Alliance Against Depression elsewhere. Today these prevention programs are continued in the EU project European Alliance Against Depression (http://www.eaad.net), which encompasses 12 partners in 11 countries (Hegerl et al., 2008).

Recent publications on suicide prevention (Department of Health and Human Services, 2012) have distinguished between *universal prevention strategies* aimed at the general population (nation, state, county, or community), *selective strategies* focusing on at-risk populations (people with mental disorders, the young, older people, members of the military, etc.), and *indicated strategies* focusing on specific high-risk groups (patients with a history of suicidal behavior).

2.4.1   Universal Strategies

Universal strategies include *health-promotion programs* – for instance, public education campaigns or school-based suicide awareness programs. Public education programs are aimed at reducing stigmatization and discrimination associated with mental disorders and suicidal behavior, which may be reasons that people are discouraged from seeking help and from sharing stressful experiences with others. In many countries, community education programs focus on raising awareness for depression (e.g., see http://ifightdepression. com/en/). Key messages generally are that depression can hit everybody, depression has many faces, and depression can be treated. A 10-year national strategy and action plan in Scotland focused directly on suicide prevention: Choose Life (http://www.chooselife. net) is linked with a national program for improving mental health and well-being, and a campaign set up to challenge stigma and discrimination around mental ill health. Some campaigns specifically focus on men. Research and clinical findings suggest that women and men differ considerably in recognizing and talking about symptoms of depression and emotional crises. Men generally tend not to recognize the typical signs of mental health problems such as depression, etc. This may be one of the reasons for the differences in suicide rates between men and women.

School-based programs, besides promoting awareness of psychological problems and depression, focus on protective factors against suicide, such as interpersonal problem-solving skills, seeking help for oneself or friends, and enhancement of self-esteem. An overview of universal prevention interventions at middle and high school levels can be found in Goldsmith et al. (2002, pp. 293 ff).

Other universal prevention strategies deal with *suicide reporting in the media* (see the Werther effect in Section 2.2.3). Studies have shown that news reports and fictional accounts of suicide in movies and television can lead to increases in suicide. Guidelines stress that media accounts of suicide should neither romanticize nor normalize suicide, and that they should include factual information on the importance of recognizing warning signs and seeking help. It is important to inform the media how important it is to present accurate and responsible portrayals of suicide and related issues (e.g., mental and substance use disorders, violence). In Switzerland, implementation of guidelines for media did have an effect on suicide reporting, and resulted in less sensational and higher quality articles (Michel, Frey, Wyss, & Valach, 2000). Similarly, Etzersdorfer and Sonneck (1998) demonstrated that ongoing cooperation with newspaper editors may have an effect not only on the quality of reporting but also on suicide rates.

Reducing availability of means for suicide includes such elements as improved legislation for firearms, installation of safety barriers on bridges, reducing access to drugs with high toxicity, and using blister packs for medications. Several studies have shown that the rates of suicide with firearms as well as the overall suicide rates are related to the strictness of gun control laws and the proportion of households owning firearms (Ajdacic-

Gross et al., 2006; Beautrais et al., 2006; Reisch et al., 2013). Changes in the availability of toxic analgesics, which have been widely used for deliberate overdosing, have had a marked beneficial effect on poisoning mortality involving these drugs, and with little evidence of substitution by other suicide methods (Hawton et al., 2004; Hawton et al., 2009). Interventions at suicide hotspots – for example, tall structures used for jumping – are another effective means of reducing suicides (Cox et al., 2013). Several studies have demonstrated that suicide rates are reduced once physical barriers are put in place, and that they rise when barriers are removed (Beautrais, 2007; Beautrais, Gibb, Fergusson, Horwood, & Larkin, 2009). Pirkis et al. (2013) showed that after a structure was secured, some increases in suicide at neighboring sites were found, but that there was an overall gain in terms of a reduction of suicides by jumping. Similar findings were reported by Reisch and Michel (2005) after safety nets were installed at the Münster Terrace of Bern.

2.4.2   Selective Strategies

Selective strategies focus on the promotion and implementation of effective clinical and professional practices for identifying, assessing, and treating those at risk for suicidal behaviors. Target groups are *vulnerable individuals* – for example, those who are suffering from mental disorder, trauma, or abuse. Selective strategies include training programs for gatekeepers (primary care physicians, school counselors) dealing with at-risk groups, such as youths, older people, members of the military, minority populations, etc. Various national campaigns have concentrated on the training of physicians in the recognition and treatment of depression. As 50% to 70% of people who attempt suicide suffer from depression, the professional diagnosis and treatment of these individuals is central to suicide prevention. The Gotland study (Rutz et al., 1989) is an example of an effective training program for physicians on the Swedish island of Gotland with a population of 58,000 (see Section 2.3.1). However, although for years the importance of recognizing depression in the prevention of suicide has been highlighted in continuing medical education (an example in Switzerland is the campaign Crisis and Suicide, 1992–1995), experience has shown that the effect of this preventive strategy is limited. In particular, depression in men continues to be severely underdiagnosed and undertreated (Rutz, von Knorring, Pihlgren, Rihmer, & Walinder, 1995; Rutz, 2010).

2.4.3   Indicated Strategies

The aim of indicated strategies is to reduce the risk of a relapse or chronicity of a medical condition in affected individuals. In suicide prevention, the objective is to improve the professional care for *individuals identified as being at risk for suicide*, in particular those with a history of suicidal behavior, given that attempted suicide is the most important risk factor for further suicidal behavior (Runeson, 2002). The National Strategy for Suicide Prevention 2012 (Department of Health and Human Services, 2012) lists a number of specific preventive elements, such as improving patient-centered care; enhancing effective therapeutic alliances; increasing resilience; developing specific clinical interventions, such as safety planning; alignment of clinical approaches with patients' needs (e.g., underlying psychiatric and/or substance use disorders, trauma support, complicated grief); immediate access to crisis services; continuity of care, including immediate follow-up after discharge from an inpatient unit; and empowerment of families and significant others in treatment, etc. (Luxton, June, & Comtois, 2013). Rogers and Soyka (2004) stressed the shortcomings of a "one size fits all" approach to suicidal patients, which is somewhat characteristic for the traditional medical model. Lizardi and Stanley (2010) pointed out the need for individualized risk assessment and stressed the importance of treatment engagement, defined as "being committed to the therapeutic process and being an active participant in a collaborative relationship with a therapist to work to improve one's condition."

ASSIP brief therapy is a typical form of prevention indicated for high-risk patients with a history of attempted suicide, specifically aimed at a patient-oriented understanding of suicidality and establishing a therapeutic alliance, which set the ground for effective safety planning.

2.5   Attempted Suicide: Psychological Treatments

2.5.1   Problems in Clinical Suicide Prevention

Between 15% and 30% of patients who have attempted suicide will show repeat suicidal behavior within 1 year (Owens et al., 2002; Schmidtke et al., 1996). Attempted suicide is the most important risk factor for suicide, with the risk being at its highest in the first 6 months after an episode (see Section 2.2.3).

So far, very few specific treatments have been able to demonstrate an effect on the risk of repetition of suicidal behavior (for reviews, see Arensman et al., 2001; Brown & Jager-Hyman, 2014; Hepp et al., 2004). Most treatment studies have had a follow-up of 6 or 12 months. Several therapy studies were unable to find an effect on suicidal behavior (e.g., Bennewith et al., 2014; Johannessen, Dieserud, De Leo, Claussen, & Zahl, 2011; Kapur et al., 2013; Morthorst, Krogh, Erlangsen, Alberdi, & Nordentoft, 2012). In view of this unsatisfactory situation, rightly, the National Action Alliance for Suicide Prevention (2014) has given the highest priority to its Action Plan Aspirational Goal 6: to "ensure that people who have attempted suicide can get effective interventions to prevent further attempts." In particular, the document states that interventions should be feasible, effective, and fast acting. This goal refers particularly to recently discharged patients – that is, to patients with a high risk of suicidal behavior.

In clinical practice, patients with suicidal behavior are known to be difficult to engage in follow-up treatment. One of the problems is that suicidality is often not addressed in the treatment of suicidal patients. For instance, Isometsä et al. (1995) found that in 571 cases of completed suicide, the topic of suicide was addressed in only 22% of cases during the last visit to the clinician. Among psychiatrists, this figure was 49%, among family doctors 11% and among specialists 6%. This may seem surprising at first, but clinicians know that suicidal people very often keep suicidal thoughts to themselves. Suicidal thoughts tend to be treated as something secret, private in the sense of "I don't want it taken away from me." The person at risk needs a special approach in order to bridge the communication gap between patient and health professional, and to talk openly about the inner turmoil and the suicidal plans.

Another aspect in the treatment of suicidal people is that following a suicide attempt, patients very often (50% or more) do not keep their appointments for follow-up care. From those who attend, more than 60% drop out of therapy after the first session (Grimholt, Bjornaas, Jacobsen, Dieserud, & Ekeberg, 2012; Lizardi & Stanley, 2010). The finding in a study in Bern, that 1 year after their suicide attempt, only 10% of patients said in retrospect that they might have consulted a medical doctor to seek help, suggests that suicidal people tend not to think that suicidality is a medical problem (Michel, Valach, & Waeber, 1994). Patients and medical professionals often have differing ideas about suicidality. The following is a statement by a 36-year-old man after discharge from a crisis intervention unit:

> What annoyed me most in hospital was being continually asked if I would do it again. They weren't at all interested in me and my feelings. Life is not so straightforward and if I'm honest, I couldn't say that I wouldn't try it again. I was sure that I didn't trust any of these doctors enough to talk openly about myself to them. (Michel, Dey, & Valach, 2001, p. 232)

The perception of help received after attempted suicide, as reported by patients, is associated with such staff attributes as sympathy and listening behavior (Treolar & Pinfold, 1993). The highest correlation between perceived help and staff attributes was related to listening behavior and sympathy toward the patients. In this study, patients preferred the possibility of emergency contacts and follow-up appointments by social workers and nurses to that of medical doctors. This may not be so surprising, because medical health professionals, when seeing suicidal patients, tend to focus on symptoms of psychiatric disorder, neglecting the suicidal patient as an individual with their motives of suicidal behavior. They are responsible for risk assessment, implementing adequate safety measures, and the treatment of the underlying psychiatric disorder. However, as therapists they should be good and empathic listeners, working toward a shared understanding of the patient's very individual and subjective experience. These two roles are radically different from each other: In explaining suicidal behavior, the patient is the expert of his or her story, while, in assessing psychopathology and deciding on treatment, the clinician is the expert.

It has been argued that the emergency department is a revolving door through which suicidal patients frequently return (Larkin & Beautrais, 2010). However, experience suggests that after a suicide attempt there is a window of opportunity for patients to be reached. Very often, shortly after the attempt, patients are open to talking about their emotional and cognitive experiences related to the suicidal crisis, particularly if the clinician is prepared to explore the intrasubjective meaning of the act with the patient. In a critical moment in a patient's life, a meaningful discourse with another person can be the turning point, in that life-oriented goals are reestablished. This requires the clinician to have the ability to empathize with the patient's inner experience and to understand the logic of the suicidal urge, even in an emergency department setting. Engaging the patient in a therapeutic relationship in a first assessment interview will increase the patient's motivation for treatment (Michel et al., 2002). Lizardi and Stanley (2010) stressed the importance of individualized risk assessment and planning of the clinical procedure in close collaboration with the patient.

ASSIP is a specific treatment program that is applied in addition to the usual clinical management and treatment of the suicidal patient. ASSIP fulfills the criteria of a therapy that can be used in clinical practice by clinicians without intensive training and that can be offered to the patient shortly after the suicide attempt. It is brief, well structured, with an emphasis on the development of an early therapeutic alliance (Gysin-Maillart et al., 2015).

2.5.2   Outreach Interventions

Reviews of treatment programs suggest that outreach elements may be especially effective interventions (Hepp et al., 2004). For instance, a 4-month outreach program, with an initial home visit to establish a relationship, followed by weekly or fortnightly contacts, resulted in a higher treatment attendance in the intervention group than in the control group (Welu, 1977). In a study by Guthrie et al. (2001), a brief psychodynamic interpersonal therapy was delivered in the patient's home and resulted in a significant decrease of self-harm in the intervention group after 6 months. Home visits in case of noncompliance resulted in a significant increase in compliance and a nonsignificant decrease in the occurrence of repetition of self-harm (Van Heeringen et al., 1995).

Telephone calls have been associated with reduced frequency of suicide. In northern Italy, significantly fewer suicide deaths occurred among older patients who were contacted by telephone twice weekly (De Leo, Buono, & Dwyer, 2002).

There is much to indicate that a form of therapeutic connectedness (or anchorage) can be helpful. This has been demonstrated by a study by Motto and Bostrom (2001), which evaluated the effect of regular letters sent to patients who had been seen in the emergency department after a suicide attempt. Out of 3,005 patients hospitalized because of a depressive or suicidal state, 843 patients who had refused ongoing care were randomly divided into two groups. Patients in one group were contacted by letter at least four times a year for 5 years. The other group, the control group, had no further contact. Formal survival analysis revealed a significantly lower rate of suicide in the contact group for the first 2 years; differences in the rates gradually diminished, and by year 14, no more differences between groups were observed. The letters read as follows:

> *Dear ...,*
> *It has been some time since you were here at the hospital, and we hope things are going well for you. If you wish to drop us a note, we would be glad to hear from you.*

A significant effect on repetition rates over 5 years was also demonstrated by Carter et al. (2005, 2013), who sent postcards in a sealed envelope in months 1, 2, 3, 4, 6, 8, 10, and 12 after discharge, while a similar study in New Zealand did not find an effect (Beautrais, Gibb, Faulkner, Fergusson, & Mulder, 2010).

A few studies have evaluated the preventive effect of a so-called green card (a card of the size of a credit card with a telephone number allowing easy 24-hr contact with a health service). Morgan et al. (1993) and Cotgrove et al. (1995) offered easy access to a therapist or readmission on demand in the case of a crisis. In both studies, there was a remarkable, albeit statistically nonsignificant, reduction of self-harm in the green card group. This reduction was independent of the actual use of the green card.

GPs can often provide a form of life-saving therapeutic anchoring. This is illustrated by the following quote from a patient:

> He [the general practitioner] was like a rock. He really was, he was genuinely concerned for me and I could tell he was. He was really worried and in a way he made me feel better you know that someone cared and he, you know, he would see me every, maybe every month every two months just to see how everything was and till he retired really so he was a great help. (Sinclair & Green, 2005, p. 1114)

ASSIP integrates insights gained from studies on interventions providing long-term therapeutic contact, by using regular semistructured letters sent to patients after termination of the four sessions, for a period of 2 years. The aim is to maintain a continuing, although minimal, therapeutic relationship, to remind patients of the continuing risk, of the importance of the safety strategies, and of how they can access professional caregivers quickly and easily.

2.5.3   Cognitive Behavior Therapy

Cognitive therapies are focused on modifying dysfunctional beliefs and behavior through cognitive restructuring. Cognitive case conceptualizations include the identification of trigger situations and negative automatic thoughts, and the emotional and behavioral consequences of these thoughts and core beliefs. The suicidal belief system is characterized by pervasive hopelessness (Rudd et al., 2001, p. 29), which manifests itself by core beliefs such as unlovability, helplessness, and poor stress tolerance. The concept of the suicidal mode (see Section 3.1.6 "The Suicidal Mode"), based on Beck's theory of modes (Beck, 1996) plays a central role in CBT of suicidality. A major goal of CBT is the facilitation of self-monitoring, self-awareness, and emotion regulation. Brown et al. (2005) evaluated the effect of CBT for people who had attempted suicide, in a randomized controlled trial. In the follow-up period of 18 months, 24% of patients in the intervention group and 42% in the control group (treatment as usual) had attempted suicide again. This treatment has been manualized (Wenzel, Brown, & Beck, 2009), but so far the study has not been replicated. The therapy comprised 10 sessions and included enhanced usual care in the form of case managers whose task was to keep in contact with patients, to reach out to those who dropped out of treatment, to motivate patients to comply with additional psychiatric treatment, and to provide appropriate referrals for further treatment. The authors stressed the importance of consulting with other health professionals and agencies for problems such as severe chronic health problems, recurrent mood disorders, substance abuse problems, social problems, etc. Clinician and patient collaboratively developed a list of hierarchically arranged coping strategies for patients to use during a suicidal crisis. Toward the end of the treatment sessions, patients underwent a *relapse prevention task* (Brown, Wenzel, & Rudd, 2011, p. 287). The objective of this task was to prime, through guided imagery, specific thoughts, images, and feelings associated with prior suicide attempts. The patients were then asked to describe systematically the manner in which they would cope with the suicidal crisis.

ASSIP, in the fourth (optional) session, includes the development of safety strategies, a rehearsal of the safety plans through reexposure to the recent suicidal crisis by use of the video-recorded narrative interview from Session 1. Patients are asked to retrieve the coping strategies that they learned in therapy to cope with the situation.

Safety planning has been recommended as a single crisis intervention strategy (Stanley & Brown, 2012). A safety plan consists of warning signs, and coping strategies patients can use without involving other people (internal strategies). These are usually behavioral activities to distract the patient from thinking about suicide. External strategies may involve relatives, friends, and other people who can be contacted for support or help in times of crisis, as well as information for contacting mental health professionals. In addition, coping cards or a Hope Kit (Wenzel et al., 2009, p. 277) can be used for safety planning (see Section 3.6.2).

Slee and colleagues (2008) used a cognitive behavior approach with adolescents and young adults, supplementing usual clinical care following an episode of self-harm. The treatment program comprised 10 weekly outpatients sessions followed by two follow-up sessions. All together, the intervention lasted approximately 5.5 months. The underlying model assumed that vulnerability to self-harm could be reduced by changing negative suicidal thinking and problem-solving deficits. The therapy focused on the exploration of the motives and reasons for the suicidal act as well as the relationship between emotional, cognitive, and behavioral factors. Therapists played an active part in keeping patients in treatment (e.g., calling patients to remind them of appointments). Nine months after initiating treatment, the intervention group showed less suicidal cognition, and less depression and anxiety, as well as an improvement in problem-solving skills and self-esteem. The authors argue that targeting cognitions of helplessness and problem solving may have been the main therapeutic effect factors.

Most CBTs for suicidality are aimed at a permanent cognitive restructuring of the suicidal mode (Rudd et al., 2001, p. 40). They require therapists experienced in the use of cognitive behavior techniques. In contrast, ASSIP does not require specific training in CBT. ASSIP therapists should have counseling experience and the skills to establish a therapeutic alliance, using a patient-oriented, collaborative approach. The objective of ASSIP is not to achieve a permanent change of the psychological mechanisms leading to suicidality or to "cure" suicidality. The aim clearly is to establish new contingent response and safety strategies for patients to apply in future suicidal crises.

2.5.4 Emotion Regulation

Most therapies developed to reduce suicide risk include interventions aimed at emotion regulation. From a neurobiological perspective, mental pain is associated with stress-induced impairment of PFC function, the brain region associated with cognitive control of emotional impulses. Therapeutic interventions aim at preventing a person from "getting lost" in the suicidal mode (which has been described as "autopilot" behavior). Interventions focus on developing strategies for early detection of warning signs, establishing alternative cognitive and behavioral response patterns, decreasing hopelessness, and on deactivating the suicidal mode by introducing and improving the skills related to emotion regulation. Safety plans rely on contingent safety strategies as a response to emotionally critical situations.

Patients with a borderline personality disorder, a typical mental disorder with emotional instability, have an approximately 9% lifelong risk of a completed suicide (Soloff, Fabio, Kelly, Malone, & Mann, 2005). Some 75% of all borderline patients demonstrate self-harming behavior, which is a predictor for later suicide. *Dialectical behavior therapy* (DBT; Linehan, 1993a), a highly specific treatment for patients suffering from borderline personality disorders has been shown to reduce the frequency of suicide attempts and hospital days, and to improve treatment compliance over a 1-year follow-up (Linehan et al., 2006). DBT basically consists of the following elements: individual therapy, skills training in groups, access to telephone contact with therapists, and regular supervision and consultations for the therapist. Therapy is organized around targets such as eliminating life-threatening behavior, reducing treatment-interfering behavior such as nonattendance and not doing homework, and ameliorating behaviors leading to a impaired quality of life such as social problems, drug dependence, etc. The therapeutic relationship in DBT is used as an ongoing expression of acceptance on the part of the therapist toward the client as well as a powerful agent for change (Rizvi, 2011). In DBT, validation strategies are crucial in reducing emotional arousal when a patient presents in a state of high distress, as is frequently the case with suicidal individuals with borderline personality disorder (Linehan, 1997). The DBT interventions consist of 16 weeks of treatment defined as 2 hr weekly skill training in groups, 1 hr weekly individual psychotherapy, and an opportunity for telephone coaching with the therapist. One of the difficulties encountered by therapists when treating suicidal patients is the feeling of being overwhelmed or even hopeless when patients have chronic or recurring episodes of suicidal ideation or make repeated suicide attempts. Peer supervision or a "consultation team" for therapists is highly recommended and is required as part of the therapeutic work. DBT is complex and intense, involving both inpatient and outpatient regimes. It is not easily implemented in the usual clinical setting in its full empirically supported package. ASSIP as a brief therapy is not suited for borderline personality disorder patients, as problems with emotion regulation clearly require long-term, intensive therapy.

Another form of therapy that showed a significant effect in randomized studies in the treatment of borderline personality disorders is *mentalization-based treatment* (Bateman & Fonagy, 2004). This therapy program has been evaluated in a 18-month and 5-year follow-up (Bateman & Fonagy, 2001, 2008) for a combination of inpatient and outpatient treatment regimes. The focus is on a gradual transformation of a nonreflecting mode of experiencing the internal world, to one where the internal world is treated with more circumspection and respect (Fonagy et al., 2004, p. 371). The capacity to mentalize is closely associated with secure attachment and the concept of the secure base (see Section 2.3.4). Both are associated with the capacity to generate coherent narratives and to maintain a continuity of the self even in turbulent interpersonal episodes.

Mindfulness-based cognitive therapy (Williams & Swales, 2004) increases patients' awareness of present moment-to-moment experience, and enhances autobiographical memory function (Williams, Teasdale, Segal, & Soulsby, 2000). The practice of mindfulness meditation has been shown to lead to measurable alterations in brain function, which are assumed to be associated with emotional stability (Davidson et al., 2003). The principle of mindfulness is derived from Zen Buddhism and is based on the premise that even in moments of crisis, people can make themselves aware of their current state – and can also develop a counterbalance to stress-driven, impulsive actions.

The close relationship between suicidality and early traumatic experiences is well established (Bruffaerts et al., 2010). Most *trauma therapies* are based on the reorganization of memories of traumatic events and their integration in the patient's life story through emotional reactivation, which takes place in a secure, therapeutic setting (Resick & Schnicke, 1993). One of the established methods is narrative exposure therapy (NET), developed by Schauer et al. (2012). The narrative of the trauma (or traumas) is central to this therapy, as is exposure to hot spots, which trigger a strong activation of the patient's trauma memory. In this way, a cognitive reevaluation and emotional restructuring is achieved. Similarly, in ASSIP, patients during their suicide narratives usually show a strong emotional involvement. In the second session, the suicide narrative is reprocessed by means of the video playback. With the case conceptualization focusing on a patient's specific vulnerability, trigger events, and the subjective experience of the suicidal mode, the ASSIP therapist offers the patient an easy to understand framework for emotional and cognitive reintegration of the suicidal crisis.

The literature on trauma therapy, attachment, mentalization, and suicide intervention converge in recognizing the therapeutic value of the narrative – that is, telling the story to an empathic listener, a key element of ASSIP.

2.6　Pharmacotherapy

The traditional medical model holds that suicide and attempted suicide are closely related to mental disorders. Indeed, almost all psychiatric diagnoses go hand in hand with an increased risk of suicide (Harris & Barraclough, 1997). As 50% to 70% of people who die through suicide fulfill the diagnostic criteria for affective disorders at the time of suicide, treatment with antidepressants is considered to be the main therapeutic component for preventing suicide (Clayton, 1983). Other diagnoses associated with a high suicide risk are schizophrenia, substance abuse, and personality disorders.

Numerous studies have shown that depression often goes undetected by health professionals, and when detected, is not properly treated (Murphy, 1975; Oquendo et al., 2002; Suominen, Isometsä, Henriksson, Ostamo, & Lönnqvist, 1998). Despite major efforts in training, the problem remains largely unchanged (Isometsä, Henriksson, Aro, & Lönnqvist, 1994). Several postmortem studies on suicide victims found antidepressants in their blood in only a minority of cases, and only rarely in an adequate concentration – that is, in spite of the strong association of suicide with clinical depression, many people who commit suicide have been taking no antidepressants or only in an insufficient dosage (Isacsson et al., 1994; Marzuk et al., 1995). The Gotland study provided a strong argument for the importance of diagnosing the symptoms of depression and their proper treatment with antidepressants. In this study, Rutz et al. (1989) instructed the family doctors on the Swedish island Gotland for two semesters on how to recognize and treat depression. Subsequently the suicide rate on Gotland fell by 60%, while the prescription of antidepressants rose by 50% to 80% in comparison with the mainland. Higher rates of prescriptions for antidepressants have been shown to correlate with decreasing suicide rates (Isacsson, 2000), but the causal relationship has been questioned. The increasing number of prescriptions for antidepressants can be interpreted as a measure of the heightened awareness of the diagnosis of depression. In spite of the strong link between depression and suicide, the evidence for the antisuicidal effect of antidepressants is not conclusive (Fergusson et al., 2005; Khan, Khan, Kolts, & Brown, 2003). Selective serotonin reuptake inhibitors can increase suicidal ideation and the risk of attempted suicides, particularly in the first 2 weeks of antidepressant pharmacotherapy (Teicher, Glod, & Cole, 1990). The danger is greater among adolescents and young adults, a finding which prompted the US Food and Drug Administration to issue a warning regarding antidepressant prescribing. However, the need for this "black box" warning is a matter of controversy (Gibbons et al., 2007).

Regarding maintenance treatment with antidepressants, various studies have shown that the pharmacological treatment of recurring depressions is linked to a lower risk of suicide (Yerevanian, Feusner, Koek, & Mintz, 2004). Angst et al. (2005) followed a cohort of people born between 1959 and 1963 for many years and showed that the frequency of suicide over 40 years was significantly lower among those patients who took antidepressants, neuroleptics, or lithium as part of a long-term therapy. The authors attributed their findings to the effect of medication, and did not take into account the preventive effect of a long-term relationship between prescriber and patient ("therapeutic anchorage"). Other authors have implicated the treatment relationship as an unmeasured but likely significant contributor to improved survival in patients. Lithium, used for long-term relapse prevention of bipolar disorder, is of special interest in suicide prevention. Studies have provided evidence that lithium has a clear antisuicidal effect (Baldessarini & Tondo, 2001; Muller-Oerlinghausen, Muser-Causemann, & Volk, 1992), even if the mood-stabilizing effect is unsatisfactory. Both suicide and attempted suicide are decreased among patients taking lithium (Cipriani, Pretty, Hawton, & Geddes, 2005).

Many patients discontinue antidepressant treatment prematurely (Olfson, Marcus, Tedeschi, & Wan, 2006). Successful treatment with antidepressants requires a close and continuous specialist supervision to ensure the evaluation and optimization of the pharmacological effect. People suffering from depression, and those close to them, must be informed that antidepressants only have a positive effect on the mood of patients after 2 to 3 weeks. Krupnick et al. (1996) demonstrated the strong association between patient–provider alliance and positive outcome in both psychotherapy and pharmacotherapy. The authors describe how this capacity for engagement may create a "holding" environment, which allows concerns to be addressed and worked through within the context of a supportive and collaborative relationship, thus enhancing the acceptance of a drug. Sabo and Rand (2000) propose a stance that puts doctor and patient in the role of "coinvestigators," in what they call "relational psychopharmacology." Even in pharmacotherapy, a therapeutic alliance should be built around principles of trust, respect, and mutuality.

Ideally, medication is one element in a comprehensive therapeutic plan that should be understandable and transparent to the patient. Needless to say, a good therapeutic relationship implies that treatment goals of patient and therapist are largely congruent (Bostwick, 2011). The patient will then see medication as a part of larger goals that include improving self-esteem through taking interest in their personal story, and providing hope that circumstances can change for the better – and that the suicidal crisis will pass.

ASSIP concentrates on the collaborative understanding of the suicidal development and the factors related to it. Psychiatric disorders often play an important part as suicide risk factors. Depression accounts for the majority of these, and in these cases the often long-term pharmacological treatment must be part of the longer term measures and objectives. The same applies to other diagnoses such as psychotic disorders, anxiety disorders, addiction disorders, personality disorders, etc. It is paramount that the ASSIP therapist can integrate these aspects into the concept of suicidality that is developed collaboratively during the ASSIP sessions.

2.7   Conclusions

The following conclusions can be drawn from the therapy studies that are relevant for ASSIP:

- A strong therapeutic alliance is essential for therapy to be effective.
- The clinician should be able to empathize with the patient's inner experience and to understand the logic of the suicidal urge.
- A narrative is key for validation of the patient's own experience and for establishing a therapeutic alliance.
- Narratives provide a means of integrating the suicidal crisis into the patient's life story through emotional reactivation, which takes place in a secure, therapeutic setting.
- A realistic aim of a brief therapy may not be to cure suicidality, but to establish new reaction patterns and safety strategies for patients to apply in future suicidal crises.
- Outreach elements such as regular letters are effective.
- Therapist continuity is important in the sense of a long-term secure base experience.
- The treatment of psychiatric disorders as suicide risk factors must be integrated into the case conceptualization.

3 ASSIP Therapist Manual

3.1 Therapeutic Concepts in ASSIP

3.1.1 Treatment Engagement: Building a Therapeutic Alliance

The therapeutic relationship is vital to effective treatment of suicidality. The best techniques applied without error at precisely the right time are of limited, if any, value when an adequate therapeutic relationship and treatment alliance does not exist.
Rudd, Joiner, and Rajab (2001, p. 13)

A major difficulty in the effective treatment of patients who have attempted suicide is *treatment engagement,* defined as commitment in the therapeutic process and active participation in a collaborative relationship between therapist and patient (Lizardi & Stanley, 2010). Suicide attempters constitute a special group of patients. They are not, like other patients, admitted to a hospital because of an illness or an accident. Their admission is the consequence of an action, which usually involves planning and decision making. Various investigators have found serious problems in the therapeutic relationship between suicide attempters and health professionals (Hawton & Blackstock 1976; Weinberg, Ronningstam, Goldblatt, & Maltsberger, 2011). For instance, suicidal patients have repeatedly been reported describing health professionals as unhelpful or even ignoring them (Hawton & Blackstock, 1976; Wolk-Wasserman, 1987; see also Section 2.5.1).

Experts agree that there is no reason to be afraid that talking about suicide with a person at risk could trigger a suicidal act. It obviously is much more dangerous when persons in crisis have no one they can talk to openly about their current situation, and when they consequently withdraw and isolate themselves. We also know that suicidal people often do not *want* to talk about their suicidal intentions. When individuals see suicide as a potential way out of an unbearable situation or an unbearable state of mind, they often keep it as something very personal, something that they don't want to have taken out of their hands. People in crisis will not abandon their suicidal thoughts for the sake of another person who is trying to talk them out of suicide. They will distance themselves from suicide once they see life-oriented goals again. We must bear in mind, however, that suicidal patients often have very low self-esteem as well as a tendency to withdraw, due to a sensitivity to being hurt by the people around them (including health professionals).

In a survey of patients mentioned earlier (Section 2.5.1), 1 year after their suicide attempt, only 10% stated that a medical doctor or psychotherapist would have been able to help (Michel et al., 1994). Half of them said that no one could have helped. This in our view indicates that a suicide attempt cannot be understood as just a cry for help.

It is crucial to understand the collaborative aspect of a therapeutic alliance as an interactive, recursive, and creative process, directed toward shared goals (Michel, 2011). As a broad concept, a therapeutic alliance has been characterized as "the active and purposeful collaboration between patient and therapist" (Gaston, Thompson, Gallagher, Cournoyer, & Gagnon, 1998). Horvath, Gaston, and Luborsky (1993) distinguished three universal aspects of a therapeutic alliance: (a) the patient's perception that the interventions offered are both relevant and potent; (b) congruence between the patient's and the therapist's expectations of the short- and medium-term goals of therapy; (c) the patient's ability to forge a personal bond with the therapist as a caring, sensitive, and sympathetic helping figure.

An early therapeutic alliance has consistently been reported to have a significant influence on therapy outcomes (Horvath & Symonds, 1991). Saltzman et al. (1976) found that ratings of alliance in the third session were most predictive of persistence in treatment. This was interpreted as meaning that, while the limited experience of therapist and client with each other at the end of the first session was generally not enough to predict the future course of events, in the third session, the viability of the therapeutic relationship was evident, with the alliance having taken root. But the finding also indicates that a therapeutic alliance can be established very early in treatment.

Two established scales for measuring a therapeutic alliance, the Vanderbilt Therapeutic Alliance Scale (VTAS; Hartley & Strupp, 1983), and the Penn Helping Alliance Questionnaire (Alexander & Luborsky, 1986) may serve as examples for some practical aspects of therapeutic alliance building. Both scales share certain assumptions, which are relevant for the therapeutic relationship with the suicidal patient. These are

1. *Acknowledgment of the patient's own thoughts and feelings.* Understanding the experience of failure, self-hate, and mental pain from the patient's perspective and communicating one's awareness of understanding requires an empathic stance.
2. *Recognition of the patient's goals and the patient's need for autonomy.* Patients have their own conscious or unconscious beliefs and goals, which need to be respected and understood. While trying to reach an empathic understanding of the patient's goal of death by suicide, the therapist should carefully probe for the client's life-oriented goals and facilitate the client's movement toward them.
3. *Working together in a joint effort.* A meaningful working alliance requires a shared model of understanding of the patient's vulnerabilities and the development toward suicide.
4. *The therapist's engagement and competence.* The therapist conveys a nonjudgmental attitude, providing a sense of safety and trust, and uses his/her professional skills in maintaining a meaningful therapeutic relationship. Patients in a suicidal crisis need someone who cares and who is not frightened by suicidal plans.

A major challenge in the therapy of suicidal patients is the therapist's skills in affectively attuning to the patient's subjective experience of an existential life-threatening crisis, and to show empathy for the patient's suicidal wish, refraining from trying to talk the patient out of it. Psychotherapy with suicidal patients may evoke strong countertransference reactions, including intense feelings of anger, helplessness, and the urge to withdraw (Maltsberger & Buie, 1974). Yet the therapist's genuine effort to understand and accept the patient's subjective experience, without attempting to change it, is crucial to the patient's capacity to explore the meaning of mental pain, which in the suicidal crisis appeared to be unbearable (Orbach, 2011). When, in a self-help group, patients who had attempted suicide were asked what would have been helpful to them before they attempted suicide, their answer was unanimous: "We would have needed someone to listen to us, who would let us talk freely, and not being afraid of suicidality."

Understanding and acceptance are essential for establishing a treatment alliance that give patients an opportunity to sustain hope in the face of unbearable anguish and hopelessness. The empathic therapist communicates verbally and nonverbally that the patient's extreme emotional experience is understandable. The therapist who validates patients in a fundamental way demonstrates the belief that it is possible to bear these feelings and to uncover nonsuicidal choices (Schechter & Goldblatt, 2011). The therapist sees and reflects the capacity that the patient cannot yet experience, and maintains hope when the patient feels hopeless about the possibility of change.

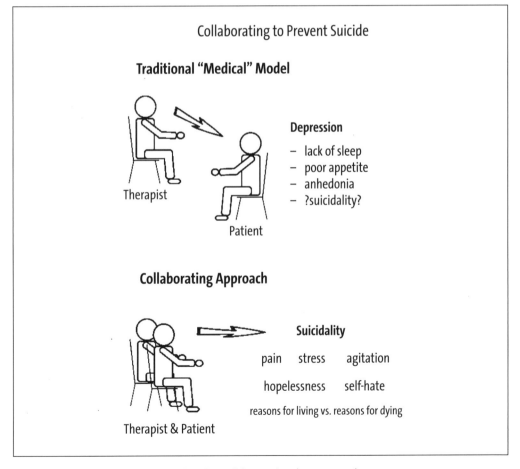

Figure 3. The collaborative approach. Adapted from Jobes (2000, p. 14).

Being empathic with the suicidal wish means assuming the suicidal person's perspective and "seeing" how this person has reached a dead end[,] without trying to interfere, stop, or correct the suicidal wishes. This means that the therapist attempts to empathize with the patient's pain experience to such a point that he/she can "see" why suicide is the only alternative available to the patient.… Instead of working against the suicidal stream and trying to instantly increase the patient's motivation to live by persuasion or commitment to a contract, the therapist takes an empathic stance with the suicidal wish and brings it to full focus. (Orbach, 2001, p. 173)

In contrast to the traditional medical approach, the ASSIP therapist uses a patient-oriented therapeutic approach, in the sense of David Jobes's "collaborative approach" (Jobes, 2006) – that is, patient and therapist *work together* toward a shared understanding of the meaning of the suicidal crisis (Jobes, 2011). In Jobes's words: "I want to see it through your eyes" (Jobes, 2000; see also Figure 3 and Box "Suicide Status Form" in Section 3.4.3). In such an approach, the suicidal patient is seen as the "expert" of his or her own life story, while when it comes to the assessment and treatment of mental health problems, the clinician is the expert. Therefore, in dealing with suicidal patients, mental health professionals need to feel comfortable in both professional roles.

3.1.2   The Provision of a Secure Base: Long-Term Anchoring

In clinical experience, safety measures such as telephone numbers and addresses of important others are usually some of the first items on the list of behavioral strategies. On their first admission to our crisis intervention unit, many suicide attempters have said that they had not been aware that they could have sought help at this address. Most likely these people will in future turn to the crisis center if the clinical care they have experienced is associated with a positive memory. Ideally, a crisis unit, therapist, or GP provides a safe place for suicidal patients or, in the words of John Bowlby, a secure base (Bowlby, 1988; see also Section 2.3.4 and the Box "The Therapist as 'Secure Base'"). According to attachment theory, in adult life attachment behavior is activated "in times of sickness or calamity" (Bowlby, 1977b, p. 428), while it may not be observable when things go well. Good clinical care must provide a feeling of security to suicidal patients, setting the necessary frame for them to engage in therapy, in which they can explore the mechanisms leading to suicidal behavior and develop individual and effective safety strategies.

Sending standardized letters or postcards to suicide attempters over several years reduces the risk of suicide, and has been explained as a form of social connectedness (Carter et al., 2005, 2013; Motto & Bostrom, 2001). In ASSIP, the authors see regular follow-up letters as the continuation of the provision of a secure base or a long-term anchoring. Obviously, even minimal offers of care can have a stabilizing effect. The results of the studies mentioned above strongly suggest that active maintenance of a long-term therapeutic connection representing a therapeutic anchoring plays an important role in the reduction of suicide risk in individuals who have attempted suicide.

In many health care systems, it is the GP that plays a crucial role in the long-term follow-up of patients, offering availability and continuity of care. The same qualities are crucial for mental health professionals involved in the care of suicidal patients. Although a personal long-term therapeutic relationship with the same clinician would be ideal, in most mental health institutions this may not be possible. In this case, easy access to a crisis team or a mental health center that people know should be provided, and patients should be informed about any changes in the responsible contact persons.

A prerequisite for a health professional to serve as a long-term secure base to a person at risk of suicide will be that the patient feels understood and experiences the therapeutic relationship as a positive and helpful experience. Therefore, a major objective of ASSIP is to establish a therapeutic relationship and a long-term anchorage in the sense of the secure base concept for suicidal patients.

3.1.3 Suicide Is an Action, Not an Illness

Considering the problems regarding the therapeutic relationship with suicidal patients, we soon realize that the medical illness model is of little help as a conceptual frame for understanding suicidal patients. Seeing suicide not as an illness but as an action, provides us with a new perspective (Michel & Valach, 1997). The action theory–based model provides a useful basis for the joint understanding of a suicidal crisis (see also Section 2.3.4). Action theory describes the nature of actions, and how we generally explain and understand actions. Human actions can best be understood in the context of hierarchically organized goal-directed systems. In an action theoretical model, life is defined by goals – that is, short-term goals that structure our day, as well as mid- or long-term goals that represent important life-career or identity issues. In this context, suicide is seen as an alternative to original life-career goals. Life-career goals may relate to relationship goals (e.g., to maintain a stable partnership) or work-related goals (e.g., to achieve a secure income to support the family). In critical times, when a person's self-evaluation is negative ("I have failed, I am a failure"), suicide may appear as a possible solution to a subjectively unbearable state of mind, and may reemerge throughout life as a possible goal in similar critical life situations. Suicide thus may become a (temporary) goal, a possible solution, when the realization of a person's long-term goals and projects are seriously threatened. The immediate goal of a suicidal action is to escape from an unbearable state of mind dominated by psychic pain, which may amount to a state of traumatic stress, dissociation, automatism, and analgesia, secondary to negative and often humiliating experience.

Here is a passage from a letter of a 39-year-old patient, written 1 year before his suicide:

> Nothing helps. I have tried everything in my life. Really, I'm looking forward to dying. My life is a series of failures in every way. I destroyed the relationships with most of my relatives and am doing the same thing with my wife. Everything wrong, always, always, always. Best wishes to everyone, to me too. I don't know where the journey will lead me but at least it does not stay in this vale of tears. (Michel & Valach, 1997, p. 214)

This man's self-assessment was "I am a failure" (something he had often heard from his father, and which thus existed as a cognitive schema) and "I'm worth nothing, my life is hopeless." These cognitions are typical expressions of the suicidal belief system (see Section 2.5.3 "Cognitive Behavior Therapy"). For him, suicide became a way of putting an end to a failed life career. He formulated suicide as a goal 1 year before his violent death. Thoughts of suicide as an alternative to life typically accompany life-career or identity crises. In *Pathways to Suicide* – still today a remarkable book – Maris (1981) in a similar sense spoke of a "suicidal career" as opposed to a "life-career."

Each suicide and attempted suicide has its individual background and individual story. Typically, patients who have attempted suicide report an unbearable state of despair, hopelessness, and the inability to see a future, a condition, which is known as "mental pain," or psychological pain (see Section 3.1.4). Mental pain is a transient and self-limited condition. Suicide appears as a solution for putting an end to a, temporarily, unbearable state of mind.

ASSIP uses the concept of suicide as a goal-directed action as a means to a patient-oriented and joint understanding of the individual's suicidality, by putting the suicidal crisis in relation to the person's important life-oriented goals. Suicide is seen as a possible solution to an adverse experience in which personal and existential human needs are acutely threatened. In an action theoretical approach the interviewer's primary task is to listen to the patient's story, and to respect patients as the experts of their own actions and as individuals with a narrative competence. This requires a definition of the therapist's role that radically differs from the role typical for the traditional biomedical model (Valach, Young, & Michel, 2011).

3.1.4   Narrative Interviewing

Every suicidal action has a very individual background. Central to action theory is the notion that actions are understood as being carried out by agents – that is, by persons who are able to monitor their thoughts, emotions, and actions, and who have, at least partly, conscious access to their reasons for why they act in such and such a way. In everyday life, we explain actions through stories, which in a therapeutic context are called narratives. A narrative is defined as a story that we tell to an attentive listener and in which we give meaning to events in order to explain a personal experience (Michel & Valach, 2011). Confiding one's own story can be therapeutic. When we are able to formulate the right story, and it is heard in the right way by the right listener, we are able to deal more effectively with the experience (Adler, 1997). Instead of ending in death as the only solution, stories about suicidal crises can open up once again the perspective of life-oriented goals.

Narratives are the means of making actions to others intelligible. The narrative is held together by recognizable patterns of events called plots. Central to the plot structure are human predicaments and attempted resolutions (Sarbin, 1986). The narrative interview therefore is not about asking why. A suicide attempt is not understood in terms of cause and effect but as an action that is embedded in an individual's biographical experiences. Normally, and for clinicians who are not familiar with the narrative interview technique, quite surprisingly, we find that suicidal patients have an impressive narrative competence. Without interference from the interviewer, a typical narrative is about the suicidal crisis, referring to recent and past events that were leading up to the present crisis. Very often, in

20 to 30 min we hear very coherent stories, in which patients spontaneously make a link between suicidality, early childhood experiences, and negative experiences later in life – for example, relationship problems. In this way, the patient and the interviewer become fellow travelers in a journey undertaken through the patient's narrative.

The Patient-Oriented Approach: The Aeschi Philosophy

In the year 2000, a small group of international experts (Michel et al., 2002) convened for a 3-day meeting in a conference hotel in the Swiss Alps, discussing person-oriented approaches to suicidal patients. On the same occasion, the Aeschi Working Group was established, which in the following years biennially organized the international Aeschi Conferences, a forum for professional exchange among leading experts in clinical suicide prevention. In 2013, these regular conferences, which attracted clinicians from all over the world, moved to the United States. The guidelines formulated by the Aeschi Working Group encompass the principles of a patient-oriented approach to the suicidal patient.

The key issues are
- The goal for the clinician must be to reach, together with the patient, a shared understanding of the patient's suicidality. It must be made clear, however, that in the working group's understanding a psychiatric diagnosis is an integral part of the assessment interview and must adequately be taken into consideration in the planning of further management of the patient. The active exploration of the mental state, however, should not be placed first in the interview, but follow a narrative approach.
- The clinician should be aware that most suicidal patients suffer from a state of mental pain or anguish and a total loss of self-respect. Patients therefore are very vulnerable and have a tendency to withdraw. Experience suggests, however, that after a suicide attempt there is a window of opportunity in which patients can be reached. Patients at this moment are open to talk about their emotional and cognitive experiences related to the suicidal crisis, particularly if the clinician is prepared to explore the intrasubjective meaning of the act with the patient.
- The interviewer's attitude should be nonjudgmental and supportive. For this the clinician must be open to listening to the patient. Only the patient can be the expert of his or her own individual experiences. Furthermore, the first encounter with a mental health professional determines patient compliance to future therapy. An empathic approach is essential to help patients reestablish life-oriented goals.
- A suicidal crisis is not just determined by the present, it has a history. Suicide and attempted suicide are inherently related to biographical or life-career aspects, and the clinician should aim at understanding them in this context.
- The ultimate goal should be to engage the patient in a therapeutic relationship, even in a first assessment interview. In a critical moment in a patient's life, the meaningful discourse with another person can be the turning point in that life-oriented goals are reestablished. This requires the clinician's ability to empathize with the patient's inner experience and to understand the logic of the suicidal urge. An interview in which the patient and the interviewer jointly look at the meaning of the suicidal urge sets the scene for dealing with related life-career or identity themes. The plan of a therapy is thus laid out.

The aim of the narrative interview is thus to invite and encourage patients to give their own understanding of the suicidal crises. We showed that after attempting suicide, in a single interview, patients rated the quality of the therapeutic relationship as significantly better when interviewers used a narrative approach (Michel, Dey, Stadler, & Valach, 2004), compared with interviewers who used the usual clinical approach. An interview in this study was considered to be a narrative when the clinician opened the interview with the words *story* or *tell* (e.g., "I would like you to tell me in your own words how you came to the point of harming yourself").

What does this mean for the therapist? A narrative approach requires acceptance and openness vis-à-vis patients, recognizing them as the agents of their own actions. Patients, on the other hand, have the narrative competence to describe and explain the subjective logic behind an act of deliberate self-harm. The shared experience (within which narrator and listener learn together about a life of pain and failure) is instrumental in reestablishing the teller's broken sense of self. The interviewer does not compete as an expert who knows more about the patient than the patient does. Instead, the interviewer functions as an interested facilitator of an injured person's life story. From such collaborative experience, it is possible for the therapist and the patient to review the past together to learn how the patient's life and the perspectives for the future have become unendurable. Empathic understanding allows the therapist, along with the patient, to grasp how suicide came to be seen as the only available solution. Only then can a therapeutic process begin.

To facilitate the patient's narrative, the interviewer should follow certain rules:

- The interview should start with the "narrative invitation," in which the clinician defines his or her role as the interested listener;
- The interviewer should not interrupt the patient's narrative but trust the patient's narrative competence;
- If necessary, clarifying questions may be asked;
- If necessary, the interviewer may probe for more details by asking open questions ("can you tell me more about ...?")
- Throughout the interview, as an attentive listener, the interviewer should acknowledge the meaning of important life experiences and their relevance for the understanding of the suicidal crisis.

3.1.5   What Patients Tell Us

In narrative interviews, how do patients describe the mental state in the acute suicidal crisis? Here are some quotations from our video-recorded clinical interviews:

> *I was devastated, I hated myself, and I couldn't stand my thoughts any more – I kind of wanted to kill them.*

> *The inner pain was so strong, I saw no other way. It was clear to me: Ending life would finally put an end to pain.*

> *I heard a negative voice telling me, "You're worthless. Because of your inadequacies you'll never make it – I've always told you so – and you won't make it again this time. You have no right to live." The feeling of bitterness, hopelessness, and desperation at that moment was so strong that I could not bear it any more, and couldn't see the point in carrying on.*

Patients' stories often are about unbearable *psychological pain* and *unbearable thoughts.* Both may emerge when patients experience their self as unbearable. Shneidman (1993) coined the terms *mental pain* and *psychache* for such conditions. He defined psychache as an acute state of intense psychological pain associated with feelings of guilt, anguish, fear, panic, angst, loneliness, and helplessness. Mental pain is usually understood as a condition in which a person's identity or psychological existence is acutely threatened, with a wide range of subjective experiences, including the perception of negative changes in the self and its function and strong negative feelings about oneself, often experienced as torment (Orbach, 2003). Here is a typical negative self-attribution of the patient quoted above:

> My life is a series of failures in every way. I destroyed the relationships with most of my relatives and I'm doing the same thing with my wife. Everything wrong, always, always, always. (Michel & Valach, 1997, p. 214)

In such an existential crisis, from which an individual sees no way out, an unbearable sense of alarm and entrapment (Williams & Pollock, 2000) may ensue. The above letter ended with: "I do not know where the journey will go, but at least it does not stay in this vale of tears" (Michel & Valach, 1997). Baumeister (1990) in a landmark paper titled "Suicide as Escape from Self," conceptualized suicide in terms of motives to escape from meaningful awareness of the self. A central element in the causal pathway toward suicide are negative self-attributions. Failures are attributed internally, resulting in self-blame and negative affect. What follows is "cognitive deconstruction," with altered time perspective, concrete thinking (i.e., tunnel vision, absence of long-term goals, suicidal plans), and rejection of meaning. Typical suicidal cognitions are described by the phrases "I am a burden to my family," "I can never be forgiven for the mistakes I have made," and "suicide is my only option to solve my problems" (Rudd et al., 2001).

Patients may say, "I had to put an end to it" or "I wanted to kill my thoughts" – in the context of an action theoretical model of suicide, these actions are typically goal-oriented: The goal of the suicide action is to find relief from an unbearable mental condition characterized by pain, anguish, desperation, and hopelessness.

An often neglected aspect of the acute crisis emerging from the patients' narratives, are *dissociative symptoms* (see the Box "Dissociative Symptoms"). This is not surprising when we understand that psychological pain has the quality of an acute traumatic experience. Here is a typical description from one patient:

> *At that moment I felt that I was outside myself. I watched the blood dripping and felt no pain. I was not afraid, and somehow, the red blood in the water looked quite nice.*

Typical descriptions of dissociative states include being outside oneself, and feeling no pain (analgesia). The level of dissociation may fluctuate:

> *I was somewhere between trance and reality. I walked through the woods for about an hour and wasn't thinking about reasons not to do it. I only thought about that later when I had found the spot. Then I started thinking: "Why am I throwing my life away?" But these were only short episodes. My feelings were confused – I was on an emotional roller-coaster. I was not myself.*

Often, after an act of self-harm, patients describe how they switched back to "normal":

> *With the last cut I got suddenly frightened. There was the sudden fear of death and the realization: what you are doing is wrong. And then I was no more outside myself. I put some cloth onto the bleeding wound and called my mother.*

Orbach (1994) argued that "the question to ask is not what causes suicide, but rather what processes or conditions enable an individual to commit the act." Patients' narratives confirm the crucial role of dissociative reactions in the form of indifference to one's own body, absence of pain and fear, and altered experience of time. Dissociative symptoms during the suicidal action may increase the risk of further suicidal behavior because then self-harm is not associated with a negative experience of pain or fear. Therefore, in a future suicidal crisis, it may again serve as a ready action plan bringing relief that is instantly available.

Dissociative Symptoms

Typical symptoms of dissociative disorder include changes in the perception of one's self, one's senses, the environment, and time. These symptoms are transient and may vary greatly in severity. Dissociative symptoms occur in connection with acute trauma reaction, posttraumatic stress disorder, acute stress reactions, and, sometimes, panic attacks. Typical descriptions of dissociative symptoms are feeling confused or disoriented, feeling numb, acting in a trance or as if in a dream, functioning in the "autopilot mode," not feeling connected to one's own body, with no sense of somatic pain (analgesia), and with altered sense of time.

Various authors have found that dissociative symptoms are common in acute suicidal crises, and that suicidal patients often describe having acted like an "automaton" (Maltsberger, 1993; Orbach, 1994, 2003; Shneidman, 1985). The connection between suicide and dissociative symptoms is not surprising, as the relation between earlier traumatic experiences and suicidality has long been recognized. Orbach (1994) argued that due to the physical alienation and analgesia, dissociative symptoms are a precondition to make bodily self-harm possible at all. In a psychodynamic model, bodily alienation is understood as fragmentation of the self, which under normal conditions constitutes a somatopsychic entity. When dissociation occurs, the patient's self literally disarticulates and reality testing fails (Maltsberger, 2004).

Neuroimaging studies in trauma research have provided evidence that traumatic experiences are stored in the neuronal networks and that the typical pattern of brain activation can be reactivated through recall of trigger situations (Bremner et al., 1999; Lanius et al., 2001). In acute traumatic stress, prefrontal cortical function is impaired due to neural deactivation, severely limiting reasoned planning and acting mindful. Interestingly, an fMRI imaging study with script-driven recall of the suicidal crisis (Reisch, Seifritz, et al., 2010) found that the pattern of neural activation in the brain of patients who had attempted suicide had obvious similarities with the neural activation in posttraumatic stress disorder.

3.1.6   The Suicidal Mode

The concept of modes explains how a suicidal state of mind can be activated from one moment to the next by specific triggers (see also the Box "The Suicidal Mode" in Section

2.3.4). Patients frequently describe the acute suicidal condition as an on/off phenomenon. The concept of the mode as been described by Beck (1996) as an "integrated cognitive-affective-behavioral network that provides a synchronous response to external demands and provides a mechanism for implementing internal dictates and goals" (p. 4). The behavioral part of the mode includes the physiological system with autonomic arousal, along with motor and sensory system activation, which orients the individual for action such as fight or flight (Rudd et al., 2001, p. 25). In the suicidal mode, the cognitive system is characterized by the suicidal belief system, with core beliefs such as feeling helpless ("I can't do anything about my problems") and being unlovable ("I don't deserve to live, I am worthless"). The affective system encompasses negative emotions such as sadness, anger, anxiety, hurt, shame, etc. In patients with a history of attempted suicide, the suicidal mode can more easily be triggered, the threshold for activation being lower in comparison with nonsuicidal individuals. Patients should learn that the suicidal mode condition is essentially self-limited, with the duration depending on stress tolerance and strategies to cope with psychological pain.

We assume that, after attempted suicide, the suicidal mode cannot be erased by therapy, because it is stored in the neural circuitry as a response to certain specific trigger situations. With a history of attempted suicide being the main risk factor for suicide, it is realistic to expect that at any time in the future, the suicidal mode may be reactivated. This leads to the conclusion that a realistic goal of therapy for patients who have attempted suicide must be to find ways of establishing effective coping strategies for future suicidal crises. The concept of the suicidal mode is easily understood by patients and can be the starting point for the development of safety planning. Patients must learn to recognize the specific warning signs and to use contingent safety strategies to respond to trigger events. These are core elements of ASSIP.

3.1.7 Summary

In the acute suicidal crisis, patients typically experience an unbearable state of mental pain. They are in an extraordinary state of mind, often characterized with symptoms of dissociation. In ASSIP, suicide is understood as an action (and not a symptom of a psychiatric disorder). Actions are explained by means of narratives. A suicide narrative is the starting point for establishing a therapeutic alliance. The suicidal mode (as an on/off phenomenon) is a useful concept for understanding the changes in the mental state that patients experience in a suicidal crisis. It is assumed that after attempted suicide, the suicidal mode as an on/off phenomenon cannot be erased by therapy. Therefore, a realistic goal of a therapy following a suicide attempt is, in close collaboration with the patient, to establish cognitive behavior schemata, including warning signs and safety strategies, to be used as a new response pattern in future suicidal crises.

- Therefore, a brief therapy should include the following objectives (see also Figure 4);
- Reaching of a mutual understanding by means of the patient's narrative;
- Establishing a meaningful therapeutic relationship;
- Psychoeducation and introduction of a psycho-biological model of suicide;
- Emotional and cognitive activation and restructuring;
- Improving self-awareness;

- Defining warning signs that precede a suicidal crisis;
- Developing action-oriented coping strategies;
- Provision of long-term therapeutic anchorage.

a. Exploring the background of a suicidal crisis with a narrative interview and establishing a therapeutic alliance;

b. Video playback for emotional and cognitive activation of the triggering mental pain condition. Important life issues relevant for a person's vulnerability are identified. Emotional and cognitive activation and restructuring;

c. Improving self-awareness through identification of individual warning signs. Establishing behavioral strategies for future suicidal crises, and reexposure to initial narrative interview.

d. Long-term contact with patients through regular letters, reinforcing the therapeutic alliance, and reminding patients of preventive strategies.

Figure 4. Elements of ASSIP.

3.2   ASSIP: The Basics

3.2.1   Objectives and Treatment Settings

The ASSIP brief therapy is designed for patients who have recently attempted suicide. ASSIP does not replace a long-term therapy but is a specific, clinical approach that aims, by means of a minimal number of therapy sessions, to elucidate the background of the suicidal crisis and to establish behavioral preventive measures. As such, ASSIP should be seen as complementing an ongoing longer term therapy. Ideally, patients are referred for ASSIP within 14 days of the initial medical and mental stabilization (see Appendix 1). Contact with the referring therapist is important so that the work done in ASSIP can be integrated into an ongoing treatment. Ideally, the referring therapist receives a short feedback communication after each session, including an assessment of the patient's current suicidality.

ASSIP can be applied in different treatment settings. It can be used in inpatient, outpatient, or day hospital settings. It is not suitable for suicidal patients suffering from psychotic disorders. These patients may act on sudden suicidal impulses resulting from delusions and/or hearing voices. In these cases, it may be impossible to work on the background of their suicidality, and insight into triggering events is often lacking. Furthermore, in our experience, patients suffering from borderline personality disorder do not benefit from ASSIP. Their condition needs an intensive long-term therapy (which usually including elements used in ASSIP).

3.2.2   Therapy Process Factors in ASSIP

A graphical depiction of the effect factors and therapeutic modules is shown in Figure 5. Central to ASSIP is the *therapeutic alliance,* which is crucial for motivating the patient to get engaged in reducing the risk of suicide. In ASSIP, alliance as measured by the Helping Alliance Questionnaire (Alexander & Luborsky, 1986) has been found to be associated with lower suicidal ideation during the follow-up period (Gysin-Maillart et al., 2015).

A key element for establishing a therapeutic alliance is the video-recorded *narrative interview,* allowing an empathic, patient-oriented understanding of the patient's story leading up to the suicidal crisis.

The *video playback* is then used to activate the suicidal mode in a safe environment and to reconstruct the patient's story. During the video confrontation, important life issues related to the suicidal crisis are identified. This process enables the *identification and restructuring of cognitive-emotional schemata.*

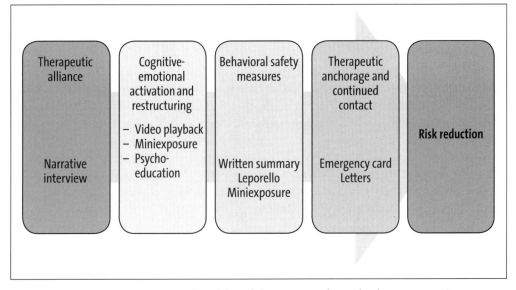

Figure 5. Therapy process factors and modules of the Attempted Suicide Short Intervention Program (ASSIP).

A *psychoeducational handout* is aimed at reaching a common, shared model of understanding suicidality. Through feedback from the patient, individual aspects can be integrated into the model.

Identification of individual warning signs in a collaborative way enables the patient to an early recognition of an imminent suicidal crisis.

Development of behavioral safety strategies is carried out jointly with the patient. A *written summary* of the background, the longer term measures (e.g., issues that should be dealt with in a longer term therapy), and the individual warning signs as well as the safety strategies for acute suicidal crises are handed to the patient. A credit card–size *leporello*[3] contains a condensed version of the safety planning.

In a fourth (optional) session, the safety strategies are rehearsed with an *exposure* to the initial video-recorded narrative of the suicidal crisis.

Regular letters over a 2-year period maintain a minimal therapeutic relationship, offering a *therapeutic anchorage* consistent with the secure base concept. Patients are reminded of fast and direct access to the professional care system.

3.2.3   ASSIP Step by Step: Overview

ASSIP usually consists of four sessions followed by continuing contact through letters. If necessary, an additional session can be offered.

Session 1. A narrative interview is conducted in which the patient is invited and encouraged to tell the story behind the suicidal crisis to the therapist. The narrative is video-recorded. At the end of this session, the patient's current suicidality should be assessed (see Appendix 4).

Session 2. Video playback: The video-recorded interview – or excerpts from it – is watched together with the patient and interrupted periodically for reflections and additional information. At the end of the session, the patient receives the written handout "Suicide Is Not a Rational Act," to be read and commented on as homework (see Appendix 3). The therapist prepares the written case formulation, focusing on the patient's vulnerabilities and suicide triggers.

Session 3. The patient's feedback regarding the homework task is discussed. The written case formulation, warning signs, and future safety strategies are completed in close collaboration with the patient. This document is handed to the patient, with copies for other health care professionals involved in the treatment and, if applicable, for significant others. In addition, the patient is given a credit card–size *leporello* with the longer term goals, warning signs, and behavioral safety strategies, together with an emergency card to ensure fast access to the health care system.

Session 4 (optional). Exposure to the patient's recent suicide attempt: The safety strategies are tested and rehearsed by watching the initial video-recorded narrative of the suicidal crisis.

---

3   A concertina fanfold or folding book, which is a long strip of paper folded like an accordion. The name originally comes from Mozart's opera character Leporello, who is the servant of Don Giovanni, the womanizer. Leporello keeps a list for his master of the ladies he has seduced. When the number rises above 100, the servant comes up with the idea of a foldable notebook and tries it out on the stairs at the opera. The name *leporello* has since then been used for foldable leaflets.

Letters: Following the face-to-face sessions, regular semistandardized letters are sent to the patient over a period of 2 years. These letters continue the therapeutic contact. They are reminders of the long-term suicide risk and the importance of the safety strategies.

3.3 ASSIP Therapy Sessions

3.3.1 General Remarks

ASSIP brief therapy consists of three to four sessions, which ideally take place within a period of 2 to 4 weeks. This time frame should, however, be adapted to the patient's mental state (e.g., severe depression) and external circumstances. Therapy session are scheduled for 60 to 90 min. Another 30 min should be reserved for case notes and, if applicable, written feedback to the referring clinician.

Important Observations

ASSIP has been devised as an add-on therapy to the usual clinical management of patients after attempted suicide. A thorough assessment of a patient's mental state, psychiatric diagnosis, and suicide risk is *not* part of ASSIP. However, the authors use the Suicide Status Form (SSF-III; Jobes, 2006) as a collaborative assessment tool that fits well with the patient-oriented, narrative approach of ASSIP. The question of the professional responsibility for suicidal patients depends on the clinical setting in which ASSIP is applied. If in an ASSIP session, the patient shows signs of acute suicide risk, the therapist has to assume clinical responsibility. In this case, the therapist would normally inform the patient about their concerns and discuss appropriate safety measures. If necessary, patients at risk should be admitted to a secure ward, if possible in the cooperation with the responsible clinician. See Appendix 4 "Assessment of Suicide Risk" and Appendix 5 "Suicide Status Form."

Many patients are eager to tell their story and are thankful for the opportunity to sit with an attentive listener who offers plenty of time to listen to them. Others are hesitant and first give a short summary of what happened, as a way of testing the ground. These patients need reassurance and validation from the therapist, who should be empathic and supportive to encourage them to open up the focus of the narrative, to give a more detailed account of what happened, and to enlarge on the biographical dimension of their story. Furthermore, patients need validation and empathic understanding for strong emotions such as shame, sadness, and desperation.

Sometimes patients do not keep their appointment or they cancel or postpone it. It is important to try to find out what the reason was, and if it was related to the last ASSIP session. It is recommended to actively contact the patient (directly, by telephone, or if necessary, by home visit). Some patients need more time to recover from a breakdown before they are emotionally stable enough to continue with ASSIP; others may need reassurance regarding the confidentiality of their therapy sessions.

3.3.2   Room Requirements

A video camera is required for the first session. Before seeing the patient, the therapist should prepare the room. Two comfortable chairs should be arranged in an angle of between 90° and 120°. The focus of the video camera should include both patient and therapist. The authors use two wall-fixed cameras, enabling a split-screen display on the monitor (patient and therapist appear on the screen in close-up and side-by-side). This technical equipment is recommended, but not essential. For the second and fourth (optional) session, a video recorder with a monitor is needed for playback. For playback, patient and therapist move the chairs so that they sit side by side when watching the video (see Figure 3).

The collaborative revision of the written materials in the third session is done on a computer, with the patient sitting next to the therapist in front of the monitor.

3.4   First Session: Conducting a Narrative Interview

3.4.1   Introduction

In the first session, a narrative interview is conducted and video recorded, in which the patient is encouraged to tell the story leading to the suicide attempt. The aim of the narrative interview is to reach a shared understanding of the individual mechanism leading to suicidal behavior in a biographical context, and to elicit specific vulnerabilities and trigger events. Narratives usually last 20 to 40 min. The session begins with the therapist giving the patients a short summary of the objectives of the therapy, even if patients have received written information about ASSIP and its structure (see Appendix 1). Basically, patients are told about the increased suicide risk after a suicide attempt and that ASSIP is a brief and structured therapy aimed at establishing preventive safety strategies, followed by 2 years of contact through letters. The therapist makes sure that the patient has understood the procedure, and asks if there are any questions. It is important to explain that the video recording is an integral part of the therapy, and that the recorded interview will be used in the playback procedure in the second and fourth session. The patient and the therapist both sign the consent form for the video recording, with a statement of confidentiality (see Appendix 6). This form is kept with the therapist's documents (see Section 3.6). Some therapists may prefer to do the introduction before entering the interviewing room, so that patients are only confronted with the video camera(s) once they have been informed and given their consent.

3.4.2   Structure of the First Session

After the introduction to ASSIP, the therapist initiates the narrative interview, making it clear to the patient that he or she is now the main protagonist:

I would like to hear in your own words how you came to the point of harming yourself. ...

In my experience, there is always a story behind a suicide attempt, and I would like to hear your story. ...

The therapist must clearly give the lead to the patient and trust the patient's narrative competence (see Section 3.1.4). As most patients are used to being interviewed in a clinical setting with the clinician asking questions, it can happen that at the start, patients relate their story hesitantly, waiting for further questions from the interviewer, but usually they soon become more relaxed and self-confident in telling their story. Some patients ask, "Where do you want me to start?" to which the therapist answers "This is up to you, you can start where you like." A common pattern is that patients begin the story with a past event ("2 years ago, my boyfriend suddenly left me, and I went through a bout of depression"), then come to the actual suicidal crisis ("I then had another relationship, but the same thing happened again, and I felt devastated and hopeless, was unable to go to work, and started thinking of suicide"), and often, without active intervention by the therapist, patients relate the actual crisis to their childhood experiences ("the story actually goes back to my childhood"). The therapist should allow patients to make pauses in their speech and not interrupt, even if certain issues remain unanswered, and important topics are only touched upon. These topics may be saved for later probing if necessary. The only questions allowed during the patient's self-narrative are clarifying questions if these are necessary for understanding the context. Note: the narrative interview is not the place for clever therapist interpretations!

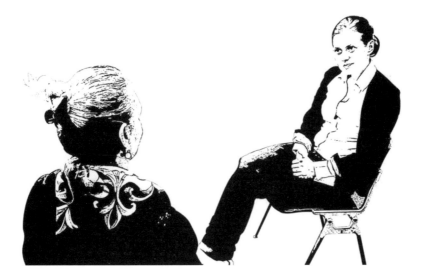

As experts of their own stories, patients should be allowed to speak freely, even if the story starts at a point which appears far away from the suicidal crisis. Only when the patient finishes his or her account should the therapist probe for more information. For this, it is important to always use open questions – that is, questions that cannot be answered with yes or no. Therapists should avoid asking why, because this is not an invitation to continue with the story but to give a short answer with no elaboration.

Examples of open questions:

Can you tell me more about this…?

In order to understand, what you mean, can you explain this to me in more detail…?

Can you tell me how the idea of suicide as a solution came into your mind?

It may be necessary to obtain more detailed information – for example, about past suicidal crises. For establishing the individual warning signs, and for developing safety strategies, it is important to know as many details as possible.

Can you tell me more precisely how that happened?

Let's imagine we were looking at how you took the overdose in slow motion….

In case the patient's self-narrative is exhausted, toward the end of the session, the therapist may take the lead in order to complete the information. If necessary, more information can also be gained in the second session (video playback). Rarely, patients who tend to ramble may need some structuring – once the therapist realizes they are getting lost in time ("May I interrupt? Watching the time, I wonder if we could jump to the moment where the thought that suicide is a solution entered your mind?"). See also Section 3.9 "Difficulties That May Arise in the Practical Use of ASSIP."

Clinical Vignette
Starting a Narrative Interview

Therapist:	Ms. S., I would now like you to tell me the story behind your suicide attempt in your own words. How did this come about?
Patient:	Where should I start? Actually the problems started at school, when I had my first crisis. At that time I didn't know what to do next, what to do with myself; it was all too much for me. I was very afraid of the future. A friend helped me through this difficult period so I got over it without harming myself. After that, years went by where I actually felt fine – until 2 years ago when my boyfriend left me suddenly, and when I made my first suicide attempt. The current crisis started in the autumn. Everything seemed to break down at the same moment. Looking at it now makes it seems ridiculous, but at that time it became all too much for me. First, the boyfriend I had at that time broke with me. That really hurt because I had thought he was *the one*. Shortly afterwards I had to go to hospital for 3 weeks for knee surgery. I was overwhelmed by the feeling that I was losing everything, and I was unable to do anything to stop it. I was very much afraid that I was completely losing control, my soul was hurting, and I felt worse and worse. But then, about 4 weeks ago, this man got in touch with me again. My friends warned me, but still, I decided to meet him. My old feelings for him were there again – until I learnt that he had been seen with another woman out dancing. Suddenly, the old pain was there again and the feeling of being treated not like a human being but like a piece of dirt. The only solution I could see was to put an end to all this. I didn't spend too long thinking about it. Last Wednesday I went to three pharmacies and collected as many pain killers as possible….

3.4.3   Ending the First Session

Towards the end of the first session, the therapist should acknowledge and validate the patient's narrative and, if possible, make reference to the patient's individual vulnerability that has emerged in the session. For instance, the therapist may say:

> *You have now given me a very good account of what got you to make a suicide attempt and the story behind it. I think I understand that in your life you have experienced many losses and breakups of relationships. I can imagine that your emotional reactions could be related to the traumatic separation of your parents at the age of eight you told me about.*

Before ending the first session it is strongly recommended to do a structured suicide risk assessment. Ideally, this is done in a collaborative way, using the Suicide Status Form (SSF-III; see the Box "Suicide Status Form (SSF-III)" and Appendices 4 and 5). The risk assessment in the first session is important for ASSIP therapists as part of their professional responsibility when dealing with suicidal patients. It is also important for the feedback to the responsible clinician. A sideline of the ASSIP sessions is that by working so closely with the patient, the therapist's evaluation of the patient's suicidality is often an important source of information for the clinical management of the patient.

The SSF is introduced to the patient with a short explanation, stating that after a focus on the patient's story, the therapist would now like to go through a set of specific questions focusing on various aspects of suicidality, to get an accurate picture of the suicide risk.

Experience has shown that the vast majority of patients, despite their emotional involvement, report that the narrative interview gave them a sense of relief. In case patients are emotionally unstable, it may be necessary to accompany them back to the ward, or arrange for a friend or family member to accompany them home. Very rarely, it may be necessary to hospitalize a patient because of a high suicide risk. This should always be done in close collaboration with the patient, the responsible clinician, and the health professional responsible for the clinical management.

We recommend that, following the first session, the therapist writes a first draft of the summary (see Box "Case Formulation and Background of Suicidal Crisis" in Section 3.6.1). This will help to expand upon unanswered aspects in the second session. It may also be helpful to make notes on specific sequences of the recorded interview that may be selected for the video playback.

Suicide Status Form (SSF-III)

The Suicide Status Form is the core assessment clinical tool used in David A. Jobes's "Collaborative Assessment and Management of Suicidality" (CAMS; Jobes, 2006). CAMS is a set of specific procedures designed to clinically assess, treat, and track suicidal risk, to desirable clinical outcomes. It builds on the primacy of the therapeutic alliance as the essential therapeutic vehicle for assessment of an individual's suicidality and required live-saving clinical care and has been evaluated in a variety of clinical settings (Jobes, 2012). A core element is the initial clinical engagement, with an emphasis on a collaborative assessment of the patient's suicidal risk. The SSF is a qualitative tool that puts the emphasis on "seeing suicidal risk through the eyes of the patient." It is a seven-page clinical tool that provides a means for the initial assessment and documentation of suicidal risk, as well as for the treatment and the tracking of suicidal risk.

In ASSIP, the authors of this manual use the first page (section A in Appendix 5) as an assessment instrument. It is applied it at the end of the first session. It needs a short introduction, explaining the importance of a more structured assessment of emotional pain and suicidal struggle. The format for this is the use of a side-by-side seating arrangement, with patients filling out the form themselves, with the therapist assisting the patient, serving as a consultant, coach, and collaborator. This procedure takes 15–20 min to complete. To compare the present suicidality with the recent suicidal crisis, the interviewer may ask the patient to first fill out the first six items of the SSF-III by recalling the very moment preceding the recent suicidal act, and then re-do the SSF for the here-and-now situation.

SSF-III sections include six items with Likert ratings (1–5) based on the theoretical work of Edward Shneidman (1987) and Aaron Beck et al. (1979), focusing on the following core aspects of suicide risk: psychological pain, stress (press), agitation, hopelessness, self-hate, and self-rated risk of suicide. This section is followed by the SSF Reasons for Living (RFL) versus Reasons for Dying (RFD) section built on Linehan's Reasons for Living Inventory (Linehan, Goodstein, Nielsen, & Chiles, 1983). This section taps the internal debate inherent in the suicidal struggle. It is followed by the Wish to Live versus Wish to Die Assessment, and the SSF the One-Thing Response ("The one thing that would help me no longer feel suicidal would be.........."). It is recommended that when using the SSF, therapists should refer to the CAMS manual (Jobes, 2006).

For the assessment of suicide risk, for the first six items, maximal Likert ratings (5) in all/most items indicate imminent suicide risk; in the RFL/RFD answers, the therapist will look for risk as well as for protective factors (e.g., family, children). In the Wish to Live versus Wish to Die section, the patient has to decide which part to score higher, while the One-Thing Response indicates to the therapist what could be a central focus in the treatment plan.

3.5　Second Session: Video Playback

3.5.1　Introduction

Ideally, Session 2 should take place within 1 week after Session 1. The *aim* of this session is for the patient and therapist to look together at the suicidal process as narrated by the patient in the first session, from the outside. This is done from an observer's position, with the patients contributing with more information and comments (see the Box "Video Playback"). In the video playback, therapist and patient reflect on the suicidal process, analyzing the suicidal process step-by-step, and identifying important life issues relevant for the suicidal crisis. The result is an emotional and cognitive reconstruction of the narrative, preparing the ground for safety planning.

Video Playback

The video playback and self-confrontation technique has been described by several authors (Hermans & Hermans-Jansen, 1995; Kagan, Krathwohl, & Miller, 1963; Young et al., 1994). Valach et al. (2002) videotaped conversations with suicidal patients and directly afterwards played the video back to them. The patients were asked to report any thoughts, feelings, and sensations they had during the interview as well as any further comments they wanted to make. After watching a sequence of 1- to 2-min duration, the video playback was paused, and the patients were asked to report. The video playback was stopped in such a way that meaningful units were provided. This technique has been used to foster reflection and induce insight into emotional and cognitive mechanisms related to suicidal behavior.

Here is what a patient wrote after a video playback:

Dear Doctor,
Since I have seen you I have been feeling unburdened. Although about a week ago I experienced again something like beginning thoughts about suicide, I do feel better than three weeks ago, after the suicide attempt. Since then I also talked more with friends, and I tried again and again to explain what happened. I feel that the interview, and above all, watching together the video afterwards, gave me very much in terms of working through. Today it is much more clear to me what a "silly" idea such a suicide attempt, or suicide itself, is.
Again, many thanks!
With best regards,
R.W.

In action theoretical terms, the video playback technique is a shared action between patient and therapist, aimed at a shared goal: to understand the suicidal crisis in a life-career (biographical) context in such a way that meaningful preventive measures can be developed. In ASSIP, the video playback allows a controlled "re-immersion" of the patient into the suicidal mode, without getting lost in it. The main goal is the analysis and restructuring of the suicidal narrative, taking an insider's as well as an outsider's position in a supportive and safe environment. This is done in a collaborative process: Sitting side by side and watching the recorded interview, therapist and patient work together at understanding the individual vulnerabilities relevant for the suicidal crisis. Video playback is thus an important part of the therapeutic process toward emotional reintegration and cognitive restructuring of the recent suicidal crisis.

In the context of the dual-processing model (see Section 2.3.4), the video playback can be seen as a situation in which the interviewer takes sides with the patient watching the narrative, which basically represents System 1 processing – that is, the suicidal mode operating automatically, intuitively, and quickly, with little or no conscious input – while at the same time activating System 2, which is associated with the conscious experience of agency, choice, and concentration. In this model, the ultimate therapeutic goal would be to program System 1 by engaging System 2, to mobilize attention when a particular pattern (warning signs) is detected (Kahneman, 2011).

3.5.2　Structure of the Second Session

First, patients should be asked for feedback from the first session. It is important to know how they felt after the narrative interview and how they dealt with the reactivation of the suicidal mode after the session. In rare cases, patients are still emotionally unstable, and the confrontation with the recorded interview may be too difficult for them. In this case, the pros and cons must be openly discussed with the patient, and it may be necessary to do the second session without video playback. Patients may be asked to talk in more depth about their feelings and thoughts, and the therapist contributes with his or her own impressions and guides the patient through the dialogue with questions.

In the second session, three goals should be kept in mind:

1. to gain a better understanding of the patient's specific vulnerability, usually seen in a biographical context (life-career issues);
2. to look at the actual suicidal behavior in detail ("like in slow motion"), if this has not been done in the first session;
3. to get some first information on the patient's own safety strategies that may emerge from the accounts of previous emotional crises.

The session then starts with the following introduction:

> *Today we shall together watch the video in which you told me your story about the suicide attempt. If you would like to comment or give me more information on a certain detail, you may stop the video at any moment, or, if I feel that I would like to hear more about a certain passage, I shall stop the video. I would also like to know how it is for you to hear your own story, and what emotions and thoughts you may have when watching it. You can also tell me at any moment in case it should become too much for you, and you want me to stop the playback.*

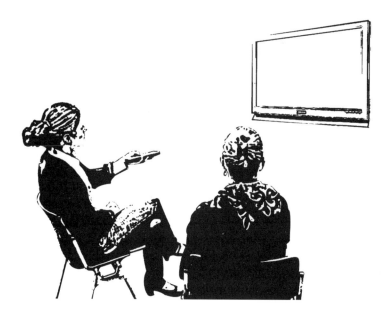

The therapist then starts the video, sitting side by side next to the patient, thus demonstrating that this is a joint action. In view of time limits and to focus on what needs to be elaborated on, it may be necessary that the therapist, before the session starts, selects the relevant sequences.

Clinical Vignette

Initiating the Video Playback

Therapist: You told me now that you felt that the session we had 1 week ago was a positive experience for you, having enough time to tell the story that ended with your suicide attempt, in your own words. Today we're going to watch the video-recorded interview together. Here is the remote control, which we can both operate. I would like you to stop the video if there is something you want to add to your story or if a point is particularly important to you. Otherwise I shall stop the video after a while, so that we can spend some time to look at some details of your story. Please also tell me if it should become too much for you, or you would like a break. Do you have any questions? If not, then I'd like to start the video now.

(After 3 min, the patient takes the remote control device and stops the video).

Patient: At that time I could only see the negative side, I couldn't see any other way and I didn't want to bother anyone with my problems. I am aware of this, that this is a pattern of mine, when things become difficult. I guess it may have to do with what I experienced in my childhood, with my parents who had no time for me. I have learnt that in life I can only rely on myself....

The therapist repeatedly invites the patient to add information, to express emotions and thoughts, also asking how it felt seeing and hearing his or her story. In close collaboration with the patient, the therapist explores and tries to identify the emerging patterns that were leading up to the suicidal crisis. Patients are asked to put themselves back into the situation again ("how did you feel, what were your thoughts?"). During the session, the therapist notes individual warning signs and the patient's own alternative action strategies ("if you were in the same situation again, is there anything that you could do differently?"). Not all patients are able at this stage to point out some of their own alternative action strategies.

What should be done with patients who don't respond to the video playback? Rarely, patients may remain passive, saying that watching the interview does not mean anything to them, that it is like watching something which has nothing to do with them. This may of course be interpreted as the patent's avoidance of strong emotions. However, in a brief therapy like ASSIP, it is not considered helpful to confront the patient with this interpretation. Rather, it is recommended to make a little "detour" in order to approach problematic emotions or thoughts. A helpful strategy here is circular questioning. The therapist may ask, for example:

Imagine that you are watching a close friend telling you this story. What would you feel about this? What would you say to him? What do you think would have helped him? What would go through your mind?

See also Section 3.9 "Difficulties That May Arise in the Practical Use of ASSIP."

3.5.3   Homework Task

At the end of the second session, the therapist hands the homework task to the patient (see Appendix 3 "Suicide Is Not a Rational Act"). Many patients experience their suicidal behavior as something that they cannot understand or explain: "I don't know how that could happen, how things could have gone so far." These patients often say that they are afraid that it could happen to them again. The therapist explains that the written hand-out contains a short text summarizing what we know about suicide and suicide risk. The therapist points out the various sections, such as mental pain, the suicidal brain, the role of early life experiences, depression, and seeking help. Patients are asked to carefully read the text at home, write down their own written comments in the spaces provided, and return the document in the next session.

The title may seem somewhat provocative, and some patients may protest against it, claiming that the suicidal act was a well-thought-out and planned behavior. The goal of the handout is not to convince the patient of the model presented in the text but to trigger the patient's thoughts about the mechanisms of the suicidal development, and to reach a shared "illness model" with the ASSIP therapist.

The main goals of this psychoeducational homework are
- to find a shared explanatory model, which can serve as a basis for safety planning;
- to foster a therapeutic alliance through the ensuing dialogue with the therapist (who must be open to the patients' arguments!).

Patients often report that the text has helped not only themselves but also their relatives to better understand suicidal behavior, and that it triggered a positive dialogue. The section pointing out the changes in brain function in the acute emotional crisis and with it the reduced capacity for problem solving often reduces self-blame and shame. Patients who experienced the acute phase of the suicidal crisis as acting as if in a trance-like state usually find the section about dissociation helpful.

3.5.4   Ending the Second Session

The therapist ends the second session by asking again how the patient feels right at this moment, how "close" suicidal thoughts are, and if he or she feels well enough to return to the ward or home. If necessary, safe transport should be organized and the responsible therapist contacted. In case the therapist feels uncertain about the patient's suicidality, we recommend adding 15 to 20 min to sit together and fill out the SSF-III. Most patients say that they experienced the reactivation of the suicidal mode through the video playback as stressful but also as a relief. Many report that looking into the suicidal crisis in detail and understanding the mechanisms leading to a suicide attempt was a positive experience.

After the session, the therapist completes the written summary with the newly gained information (see Box "Case Formulation and Background of Suicidal Crisis" in Section 3.6.1).

3.6 Third Session: Formulating the Patterns Leading to the Suicidal Crisis

3.6.1 Introduction

The main goal of this third session is to complete the written formulation of the individual processes and patterns involved in the development of the patient's suicidal crisis, as well as a list of safety strategies for the prevention of future suicidal behavior. It is recommended that a first draft of the text is written after the first and second session, by using information (notes, video) from the narrative interview and the in-depth exploration from the video playback. This draft will now be revised in close collaboration with the patient. The document which the therapist brings to the third session includes:

- A case formulation of the *background* of the suicidal crisis, with an emphasis on *personal vulnerabilities and trigger events;*
- A draft of *helpful mid- and long-term goals;*
- A draft of individual *warning signs* that precede a suicide attempt;
- A draft of individual *safety strategies.*

Case Formulation: Background of the Suicidal Crisis

The case formulation is a written summary reflecting the story told by the patient, trying to convey the logic of the patient's suicidal crisis, based on relevant life-career/biographical issues related to the suicidal crisis. The formulation should point out *individual vulnerabilities*, which in the future may again be the reason for a suicidal crisis. *Specific trigger events* related to the patient's vulnerability will be needed for activating the suicidal mode, in particular when a past suicide attempt has left a contingent behavioral response pattern. For example, a deep routed sensitivity to rejection may repeatedly be associated with negative cognitions about oneself. A serious relationship problem can then be the triggering event for a suicidal crisis. In action theoretical terms, suicide may appear as a solution when important life-career issues (goals and needs) are seriously threatened (see Section 2.3.4 "Psychological Models"). The related biographical issue in the above example would be the need for security in close relationships. Adverse experiences related to an individual's emotional needs trigger typical cognitive schemas ("I'm worthless, unlovable, I'm a burden for others; things will never change"), often representing the last step to the suicide action (see Section 2.3.4 regarding the cognitive behavior model of suicide).

The therapist has gained most of the relevant information for the case formulation in the two previous sessions: the narrative interview and the video playback.

When writing the case formulation, the therapist may be guided by the following key questions:

- What outer event and/or inner experience triggered the current suicide attempt?
- What past events (past emotional and suicidal crises, negative childhood experiences) are related to the patient's vulnerability?
- What factors had a moderating effect on the suicidal development of events (e.g., significant others, psychiatric disorders, substance abuse, ambivalence, etc.)?

- What would have to happen again, or what would the patient have to experience again in the future that could trigger another suicide attempt? The individual vulnerabilities and life-career issues mentioned above are key here. They could be the focus of a longer term psychotherapy, which will often be recommended by the ASSIP therapist (see helpful long-term measures in Section 3.6.2).

See also Section 3.9 "Difficulties That May Arise in the Practical Use of ASSIP."

Clinical Vignette
Vulnerability and Trigger Events

Patient:
The past few months have been very hard for me. I couldn't cope with how my boyfriend broke up with me.... One day I came home and he had left, taking all his belongings with him. He didn't bother to leave a message. In the following days I tried to contact him, but he didn't answer the phone ....

I didn't go to work any more, stayed at home, didn't bother to eat, or shower. From my workplace, nobody made any attempt to contact me. I was devastated. Life had come to a stop. I then decided to take a taxi and went to his apartment. He was not at home, but, as I still had a key, I went in, and I found that he had done away with everything related to me, gifts, clothes, etc.... This triggered the suicidal crisis. I got into such a strange state of mind, acting like a zombie. I knew where he kept the pain-killers, I found two packages, with some 20 tablets each, and I then took the whole lot, left the place and went to the river. I wanted to die. My thoughts were: There is no use, things will never get better.

I know this feeling of being left alone, of being treated like dirt, without explanation, from earlier experiences in my life; it happened with my mother, many times, and already then I thought of jumping from the window. It happened in two serious relationships, one of them lasting 3 years, and they ended the same way. This was when I made my first suicide attempt, 2 years ago. I was admitted to the psychiatric hospital at that time, but I had no follow-up treatment. I often think that I am not made for this life, that there is no place for me in this world.

3.6.2   Structure of the Third Session

Review of Homework Task

The therapist starts the session by asking how the patient feels at this moment and how he or she felt after the last session. The therapist then reviews the homework task with the patient. The therapist asks for some feedback – for instance, if the patient felt that the text meant anything to him or her, if there was anything that seemed particularly relevant, and if there were any questions. It is recommended to take a few minutes to go through the text, section by section, commenting on the notes the patient has made. It is extremely important that the therapist tries to understand the patient's objections, if there are any, and to validate the patient's personal experience. In case the patient has not made any notes or did not bring along the handout, the therapist may nonetheless take the patient through the text by highlighting the main issues and hand another copy to the patient. However, if a patient is not keen on fulfilling the written homework task, it may be better not to insist.

Case Formulation

Prior to the session the therapist has made a draft of the case formulation ("background"; 1/2 to 1 page), followed by a preliminary list of helpful long-term measures, warning signs, and the safety strategies for acute crises. The case formulation can be written in the first or third person (see Box "Text Template"). We usually prefer the first person, as this underlines the fact that the summary should primarily be the patient's own story. This document will now be reviewed, revised, and completed in a collaborative manner between patient and therapist (see Case Examples 1 and 2 in Appendix 7).

Text Template

Attempted Suicide Short Intervention Program (ASSIP)

Patient's name:

Dates of ASSIP sessions:

Dear Mrs./Mr. ...,
As discussed, here is my attempt at summarizing the main points from our conversations on the background of your suicidal crisis. The following text is written in the first person, as it is your story. (or The following text is addressed to you because it is the story as I heard it from you.)

1. Background (1/2 to 1 page):

_____

_____

_____

_____

_____

_____

_____

_____

2. The following measures are important for my safety in the future:

Helpful long-term measures:

_____

_____

_____

Warning signs:

_____

_____

_____

Safety strategies against suicide:
First:

1. _____

2. _____

3. _____
Acute:

1. _____

2. _____

3. _____

Established together on (date): _____

Approved:

_____

Signature patient

_____

Signature therapist

Copies: Family doctor, psychologist

Patient and therapist sit at the table, side by side. It is important that the patient has an active role in this process, and that the final document feels right for the patient. The therapist explains the aim of this session, with the following words:

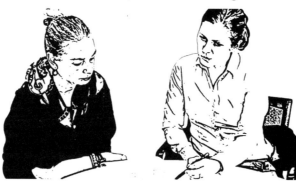

I have tried to write down the background of your suicidal crisis from what you had told me in the previous sessions, as well as some possible safety strategies for the future. Today I want to work with you on this document, so that we both know that it feels right for you. I shall read the text to you, and I want you to comment, add or delete things.

Clinical Vignette

Example of Case Formulation by Therapist

Dear Mrs. C.,
As discussed, here is my attempt at summarizing the main points from our conversations on the background of your suicidal crisis. As it is your story, the text is written in the first person.

Background
What triggered the suicide attempt: *It was when I realized that my boss would find out that I was the one who had made the accounting error. It was especially hard because I knew that I would have to face the consequences. Up to then I had managed to put it to the back of my mind. I went on vacation with my sister and paid for everything. But I was afraid I was going to lose my job, and be reported to the police. Above all I was ashamed – me, who was always so conscientious and reliable.*

I realized that everyone would now know that I had been pretending to be someone I wasn't. My pack of lies was about to collapse. I couldn't see any other way out than putting an end to my life because I couldn't stand the humiliation, couldn't stand losing face and was afraid of it. Suicide seemed the only way out. On 4.6.2014 I drove to a remote part of the wood and took tablets. Luckily, enough time went by, and I suddenly realized that my family needed me.

I know that I have this need to appear to the outside world better than I really am. Already as a child I tried to do everything so that the others didn't notice my weaknesses and shortcomings. It is like a house of cards with its walls always close to tumbling down. I also have this tendency to join in with everything, all kind of events and social occasions. I am a person who does get herself involved with everything and who doesn't pay much attention to her own needs. Maybe it has to do with my need to be accepted by others.

The joint reviewing of the case formulation can be done with handwritten notes on the printed text, or the reviewing may be done directly on the computer, with therapist and patient sitting in front of the monitor.

Once the first part of the written summary on the background to the suicidal crisis is completed to the patient's satisfaction, the therapist moves on to the second part: the formulation of long-term measures and objectives, individual warning signs, and safety strategies. Each section should comprise a list of 4–6 keywords. The list should be kept short, so that it can be copied and pasted into the Hope Leporello (see Box "Hope Leporello").

Helpful Long-Term Measures

Long-term measures include individual goals that are indirectly linked with the suicide attempt. Some examples are relationship counseling, individual psychotherapy, therapy for alcohol problems, treatment of depression or anxiety disorders, looking for a new job, etc. It may be that some of these issues emerge during the first two sessions. The therapist should encourage the patient to work on these issues as they are related to the suicide risk. If a patient is not in any professional treatment or counseling, the therapist may suggest names and addresses of therapists.

Prompting questions may be:

- We have now seen how things developed, leading to a suicide attempt. What would be helpful in the long run to reduce the risk of future suicidal crises?
- How important do you think is psychiatric treatment?
- How important is medication?
- What would be treatment goals for psychotherapy/counseling?

Example of a response: *I often get involved in other people's problems, far too much. I need to learn how to let the people around me know when I am not well. Even now I find it really difficult to do because I don't want to be a burden to anyone. Although I now know that I have the right to do it, I still have to work on it.*

The keywords for this patient are:

- Learn to recognize limits;
- Improve self-awareness: How do I feel right now? What is bothering me right now?
- Learn to ask for support from others;
- Continue seeing a psychotherapist.

Example of Important Measures for Future Safety

Helpful long-term measures:
- Improve self-awareness: How do I feel right now?
- What is good for me, and what is not?
- Resume psychotherapy
- Continue antidepressants
- Improve housing situation

Warning signs:
- Loss of appetite
- Problems with sleeping
- Circular thinking
- Withdrawing, not talking
- Negative inner dialogue: It would be better if I were no longer here
- Excessive alcohol consumption

Safety strategies against suicide:

First:
1. Go running
2. Petting the cat
3. Cook something special
4. Listen to favorite music
5. Call or visit friends, parents, brother, or sister

Acute:
1. Call my outpatient therapist (phone number: ....)
2. Call ASSIP therapist (phone number. ...)
3. Call crisis intervention clinic where I am known (phone number. ....)
4. Take a taxi to the emergency department

Warning Signs

The patients should get to know their own personal warning signs that precede a suicidal crisis so that they can recognize dangerous situations early on and react to them. This is a key aspect of ASSIP, as we work on the premise that after attempted suicide, the patient cannot be "cured" from suicide risk, but what we can do is increase the patient's awareness for future critical situations. Warning signs are extremely individual in character. They may include cognitions, body sensations, and situations. To be effective in stressful situations, they should be as specific and accurate as possible.

Prompting questions may be:
- What are your own, individual warning signs that tell you it's getting dangerous for you?
- In the recent suicidal crisis, what were the first signs of the crisis?
- In case you got into the same situation again in the future, what would be the first signs of danger?

> Example of a response: *My body reacts first. I can hardly eat anything and my sleep becomes worse and worse. I lie awake for hours and during the day feel exhausted with no motivation, and I have to force myself to do anything. Then my thoughts start going round in circles, and I start to drink more alcohol. The depressive phases always began like that. Actually I know that I shouldn't wait and that I should contact my doctor. When it gets so bad that I can't take my mind off it, then it gets dangerous. Everything in these moments is too much for me, I feel unable to cope, and I don't know how to carry on. I withdraw from everyone!*

The warning signs in this case example are:
- Loss of appetite
- Problems sleeping
- Circular thoughts, ruminating
- Alcohol consumption
- Depressed mood
- Social withdrawal

The therapist makes a list of the main warning signs, in the form of keywords that can be copied into the Hope Leporello (see Box "Hope Leporello").

Safety Strategies for Future Suicidal Crises

Here, individual strategies are developed to help the patient to stop the further progression of the suicidal crisis to a stage where control becomes difficult, such as getting in an autopilot or trance-like state (suicidal mode, dissociation). Strategies are usually cognitive and behavioral. They may include physical activity (running), playing with a pet, doing household chores, playing an instrument, etc. Cognitive strategies may be reading, writing a diary, doing crosswords, puzzles, etc. Some patients have had training in the use of mindfulness exercises. It is important that the strategies are as specific and as personalized as possible. Many patients know from earlier suicidal crises what in their case has proved to be helpful. The strategies are developed together with the patient and put into order of importance. The safety strategies can vary immensely from patient to patient. Obstacles and difficulties in the practical use of safety strategies should be addressed – for instance, the availability of contact persons.

Prompting questions may be:
- What have you used in the past to stop you from harming yourself?
- Put yourself again into the situation where you felt devastated, thinking of suicide. What could you have done to stop yourself from losing control?
- Is there anything you can use on your own?
- Where can you turn to when the suicidal impulses are becoming acute?
- How available are these people?
- Can you reach them at night?
- How much trust do you have in them?
- Can you inform them that you may need them in the future?

First (Own) Strategies

The first strategies are those that patients can employ themselves, such as going running, taking the dog out for a walk, lying down and petting the cat, taking a shower, listening to loud music, playing an instrument, doing crosswords, cleaning the bathroom, cooking a special meal, etc.

Strategies in Case of Acute Danger

In a second paragraph, strategies in case of acute risk of suicide usually involve other people (private or professionals). Examples are call a friend or a family member; go to a neighbor; call the GP or the psychiatrist; call the ASSIP therapist, the outpatient department, or the crisis line; go to the emergency department of the local hospital, etc.

Now the written document can be finalized and printed. Patient and therapist both sign it, thus giving the document an "official" contractual character. This contract also addresses the role of the ASSIP therapist in future crises, depending on availability and continuity. Ideally, in case of a crisis, the ASSIP therapist can be reached. Patients get one copy for themselves, with additional copies for health professionals involved in the treatment. Copies may also be sent by mail.

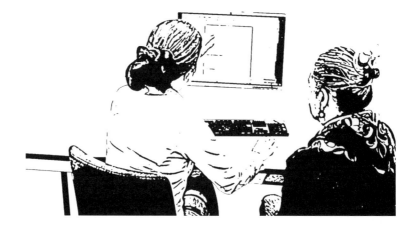

Hope Leporello

The long-term measures, warning signs, and safety strategies are now copied into the template of the Hope Leporello (see Box "Hope Leporello" and Figure 6), by copy and paste. The leporello, when folded, is the size of a credit card and can be kept in a wallet. Like this, patients have access to their individual strategies in dangerous moments.

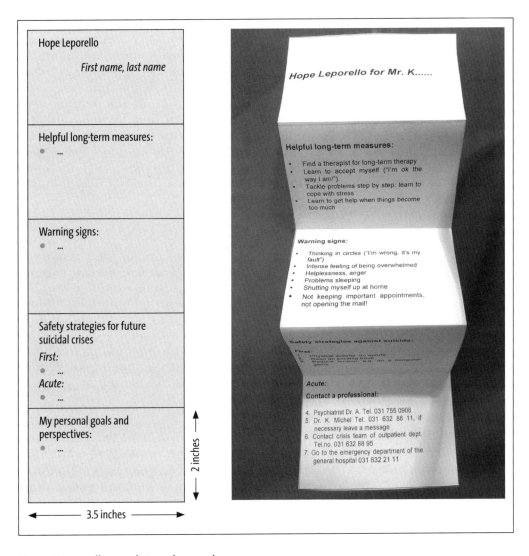

Figure 6. Leporello template and example.

Hope Leporello

The Hope Leporello contains the list of longer term measures, warning signs, and strategies to be used in case of a suicidal crisis. In addition to the safety strategies, it is recommended to use the last section of the leporello for goals and perspectives in the patient's life, in the sense of Reasons for Living (see Appendix 5 "Suicide Status Form (SSF-III)").

It is easiest to use a Microsoft Word template with an appropriately sized frame, using a font size of 8 to 10, depending on the space available (see Figure 6). A colored paper may be used, with the patient choosing the (his/her) color. The printed leporello is cut out with a pair of scissors or a paper cutter and folded along the lines to the size of a credit card. We recommend saving the leporello electronically under the patient's name (together with the other written documents). This makes it possible to revise the content at a later contact with the patient (e.g., with emergency numbers of important contact persons). Many patients ask for the leporello to be sent to them by e-mail. Some patients use the electronic form to increase the personal meaning – for instance by putting a personal picture (of a close person, a pet, a holiday picture, etc. – i.e., life-oriented contents) on the top page.

Excursus: Hope Box

In the case of an ongoing psychotherapy – for instance, in the treatment of a borderline personality disorder – the leporello can be complemented by an emergency, or hope box. Wenzel, Brown and Beck (2009, p. 277) suggested the use of a "Hope Kit" as an initial step in the crisis response. The concept of the hope or emergency box has been used in dialectical behavior therapy (DBT), developed by Marsha M. Linehan to treat patients with borderline personality disorder (Linehan, 1993b). Skills training is part of this holistic concept, aimed at improving stress tolerance and emotion regulation. Patients are asked to prepare a hope box (or emergency box), in which they place objects representing the main strategies of stress tolerance skills. The goal is that even in a state of great distress and agitation (with reduced access to cognitive strategies), patients can fall back on the resources they have learned. As a means of emotion regulation in critical moments – that is, when rational thinking is no longer possible due to extreme arousal – the hope box can be very effective.

It is important to include real objects and to keep the hope box at hand. Other content (e.g., telephone numbers) can be written on a piece of paper. Commitments and agreements with others should also go into the hope box. Some objects may have a symbolic meaning, such as doll shoes to prompt the patient to put the shoes on and go to a particular place, a toy cell phone together with a list of telephone numbers, soap to prompt the patient to take a warm bath, etc. The objects should have an emotional significance to be effective against the "autopilot" suicidal mode condition. Cognitive responsivity is limited in this state of mind. The emergency box is not part of ASSIP, but can be a meaningful addition as part of a longer term therapy. Including personally relevant and life-oriented pictures on the leporello is in line with this concept.

Emergency Card (optional)

Patients may also be given a crisis card (see Figure 7). The crisis card assures direct access to a patient's helper system and basically contains important names and phone numbers. Here too the patient is asked to carry the card at all times (e.g., in his wallet or diary).

Always carry this card!	***Important in event of threatening crisis:***
....	– Recognize danger early!
....	– Use Hope Leporello
....	– Talk to a helpful person (friends and family etc.)
	– Call *family doctor / surgery*, Tel.
	– Call Crisis unit
	Daytime Tel.
Tel. number clinic/surgery	Night and weekends Tel.

Figure 7. Example of an emergency card.

3.6.3   Ending the Third Session

The therapist insures that the patient is mentally stable. In case a fourth session (mini-exposure) is planned, the therapist asks the patient if he or she feels ready for a rehearsal session, to test the usefulness of the safety strategies. If the patient is unstable, the reexposure to the recent suicide attempt may not be advisable. In this case, the therapist tells the patient about the regular letters and explains the rationale (see Section 3.8). It is important to check that address, phone number, and e-mail address of the patient are correct. It is recommended to record the name of a possible contact person in case of change of address or phone number. If the patient has no questions regarding the next steps, the therapist ends the session.

3.6.4   Decision to Hold a Fourth Session

The ASSIP brief therapy was originally developed and evaluated with the three sessions described above. Over time, the authors decided to add a fourth session. This idea based on the work of Gregory Brown and others (Wenzel, Brown, & Beck, 2009), who used role play for the rehearsal and reinforcement of the safety strategies. We introduced a fourth session using the video from the first session (the narrative interview) as a kind of miniexposure. Clinical experience has shown that many patients greatly benefit from this technique. In addition, it is a test of the usefulness of the safety strategies as developed in Session 3. It is not rare that after the exposure, the Hope Leporello needs to be revised.

3.7   Fourth Session (Optional): Reexposure

3.7.1   Introduction

The aim of this last session is to practice the strategies developed. For this purpose, a miniexposure is conducted with the patient, using the video-recorded narrative interview. The idea is that the suicidal mode is reactivated, and that patients should explicitly indicate at which point in time and with which strategies, they would now be able to stop the suicidal process.

Exposure in Cognitive Behavior Therapy

In cognitive behavioral therapy, to establish new behaviors, old patterns, which are often related to avoidance behavior, should be reactivated. For this to happen, patients are exposed to situations which are specific, threatening, and frightening for them. To establish new coping strategies, it is essential that this takes place in a context that is motivationally and emotionally positive (Grawe, 2004). These conditions are normally fulfilled in the fourth ASSIP session: The narrative interview, video playback, and collaborative development of the biographical background of suicidal crises and the individual coping strategies create a therapeutic relationship that is characterized by a shared view of the problem and cooperative motivation and purpose.

Brown et al. (2005) in their cognitive behavioral treatment, used role-play to expose patients to the suicidal crisis after an average of 8 to 9 therapy sessions, as a relapse prevention task (Wenzel et al., 2009, p. 200). With verbal instructions consisting of guided memories, patients are guided back to the situation of the last suicidal crisis (suicide mode) and are encouraged to use the specific coping strategies. In ASSIP, the reactivation of the suicidal mode is done with the help of the video-recorded narrative interview from the first session. The advantage of this is that activation is achieved more easily, and if necessary, the corresponding video sequence can be replayed several times. Patients can stop the video themselves and indicate which safety strategy they would use at which moment of the suicidal crisis. This provides patients with an opportunity to practice their suicide management skills in a safe environment, before applying them in a state of distress. Sometimes, in the course of the session, it may be found that the strategies developed in the third session have to be revised.

3.7.2   Structure of the Fourth Session

As a standard opening, the therapist begins the session by asking about feedback from the last session and whether there is anything to add or say about the written material. The therapist then explains the procedure of this session to the patient in the following way:

> We are now going to watch the video with your story again. I would like you to put yourself back into that situation, as best as you can. What were you feeling, what thoughts did you have? Then, as we proceed, please tell me when exactly you would now use one of the strategies that we worked out in the previous sessions, in order to stop this dangerous situation.

Sometimes patients let the video run without interrupting or mentioning one of the strategies. In this case, the therapist should explore the reason together with the patient. It may be that the strategies developed have to be adapted (e.g., "I realize now that the strategy we put down in the Hope Leporello is not useful; I would have to take my cell phone *immediately* and call the hospital"). Often patients realize that they should have done something at a much earlier point in time:

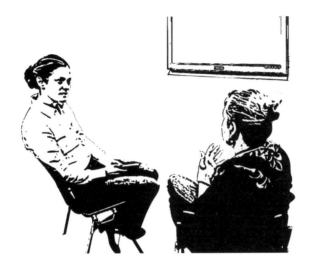

I've just noticed that it was already too late that morning. I couldn't have stopped the process, it was an automatism. I should have spoken to my therapist a week earlier. I should have told her that I was worse and I definitely should not have returned home alone after the argument with my brother.

3.7.3   Ending the Fourth Session

Before ending the session, the therapist insures that the patient is mentally stable. The therapist informs the patient about the regular letters and explains the rationale (see Section 3.8.2 below). It is important to check that address, phone number, and e-mail address of the patient are correct. It is recommended to record the name of a possible contact person in case of change of address or phone number. Patients should know how and when they can reach the ASSIP therapist, and what to do if the therapist is not available. The patient should have fast and direct access to the system of help at all times. If there are no further questions, the therapist ends the session, and with it the face-to-face interventions of ASSIP.

3.8   Ongoing Contact by Regular Letters

3.8.1   Introduction

Over a period of 2 years, patients will regularly be sent standardized letters – in the first year every 3 months and in the second year every 6 months. The letters can be complemented with a personalized sentence (see Appendices 8–13). As discussed in Section 2.5.2, several studies (Carter et al., 2005, 2013; Motto & Bostrom, 2001) have indicated that this outreach element may be effective in reducing the suicide risk. In ASSIP, the aim of the letters sent and signed by the therapist is, on the one hand, the maintenance of a therapeutic anchoring in the sense of a secure base (see the Box "The Therapist as 'Secure Base,'" in Section 2.3.4) through regular contact with the patient. On the other hand, in the event of another suicidal crisis, the ongoing contact with the ASSIP therapist insures that patients have easy access to professional help. However, a fundamental element may be that with these letters, patients are repeatedly reminded that a heightened risk after attempted suicide will remain and that they should always be on their guard.

3.8.2   Procedure

In the last session, the patients are informed that from now on they will regularly receive letters for a period of 2 years. The rationale should be explained to the patients, pointing out that a number of studies have shown regular letters can reduce the suicide risk after attempted suicide (see Section 2.5.2).

The patient should be told that:

> *From now on you will receive letters from me every 3 months in the first year and every 6 months in the second year. This is to remind you that suicidal crises can also occur in the future and that you mustn't forget the strategies we worked out together.*

Patients often give feedback via e-mail on how things have been going in the meantime. For the letter following such feedback, we strongly recommend adding a personal remark to the standardized text (often referring to the strategies developed or the feedback received). This can be done with little effort.

3.8.3   Administration of Correspondence

To help the therapist in charge to be reminded when the letters are due, the creation of an electronic database is recommended (e.g., in the Microsoft Access program). The relevant data (name, sex, contact details, number of suicide attempts, dates of ASSIP sessions) can be entered in the database. The variable for the last contact should be the starting point of the regular letters. In this way, the ASSIP therapist will receive automatic reminders, indicating the dates letters are due for each patient, and which letter (1–6). (See Appendices 8–13 for examples of standardized letters 1–6. Naturally, therapists are free to adapt the letters.)

Correspondence Template (Example)

Dear Mr. W.,

Six months have passed since your last appointment with me. I hope you are well. You receive a few lines from us several times a year because we know that even a long time after a suicidal crisis the danger is never completely gone.

Remember that even in a situation that appears at the time to be unbearable, you can pause for a few minutes, take an observer's look at your feelings, thoughts, and body sensations from a neutral position. Try to accept what you perceive ("At the moment that's just how it is. It is neither good nor bad"). Pain, mental pain, does not last forever. Suicidal impulses subside after a certain time. Wait until you feel that the level of agitation goes down.

Use the Hope Leporello we have developed together.

It often helps to talk to someone, to put things into perspective again. Don't forget that you can get in touch with us at any time. In case I am not available, please ask to be put through to our emergency team or emergency doctor (<<Tel. No.>>), they are available 24 hours.

I would be pleased to hear from you if you would like to write a few lines, but you are not required to do so.

You will receive a next letter in 3 months' time. If you no longer wish to receive our letters, please let me know by phone or by email.

Best wishes,

<<Therapist's name>>

<<E-mail address>>

3.9 Difficulties That May Arise in the Practical Use of ASSIP

Since the publication of the original manual (in German), we have gained further practical experience, above all from the training and supervision of health professionals who began to work with ASSIP. So far (autumn 2014), ASSIP has been used in clinical practice by institutions in Switzerland and Finland. The team of the Finnish Mental Health Association started with ASSIP in summer 2013. Since the introduction of ASSIP in the outpatient department of the University Hospital of Psychiatry in Bern, Switzerland, in 2009, and the publication of this manual, we have used ASSIP for over 300 patients who had attempted suicide. During this period, other therapists joined our team, and through them, we learned about some of the difficulties and practical aspects that may be relevant for new users.

Generally, new therapists have found ASSIP easy to use. Many of them reported that the clear structure of the sessions was very helpful. This was thought to be particularly important in view of the frequently prevalent feeling of helplessness vis-à-vis an individual's suicidality. It was also noted that for many patients who in the past had been treated after attempted suicide, the briefness of ASSIP and clearly structured sessions were attractive and helpful to foster treatment motivation. Related to this is the usually very small number of patients dropping out.

Narrative Interviewing

Narrative interviewing requires the internalization of a therapeutic approach based on (1) the notion that the patients are the experts of their story and on (2) the trust in the patient's narrative competence. For this it is important that therapists have a good knowledge of the patient-oriented philosophy of the ASSIP approach (see Section 3.1), which radically differs from the usual clinical practice based on the standardized assessment of risk factors, mental state, and psychiatric diagnosis.

Problems that may arise as follows:

- The patient gives a 3-min account of what happened and stops there. The therapist's intervention in this case may be: *"Okay, you have now given me a short account of what happened. Now, let's look at it in more detail. In my experience there is always a personal story behind a suicide attempt."* The therapist prompts for a more detailed account with open questions: *"Can you tell me more about…"; "can you help me understand…"* For the formulation of safety strategies, interviewer and patient will also need a very detailed account of the whole suicide action sequence (from thought to plan, to preparation, to actual suicide action, including signs of ambivalence in cognition and affect, etc.). A very detailed account is crucial, because this will give valuable information about moments where the suicidal process could be stopped. It may be helpful to tell the patient that *"in order to look together in detail at what happened, let's imagine that we both look at it in slow motion.…"*

- The patient says that he or she would rather have the interviewer asking questions. Therapist intervention: *"This is what most people are used to in an assessment interview. However, we think that by asking questions you only get answers, but not the personal story behind a suicide attempt. Try to start wherever you want. Don't worry, if necessary I will help you."*

- The patient gets very emotionally activated; some patients with a history of trauma may start to dissociate during the narrative interview. Therapist skills that may be applied here include: To interrupt the story, show empathy with the patient's affective state, take an outside view by asking the patient to comment about his or her reaction when telling the story. Patient and therapist should try to understand what is most upsetting for the patient, and what the stressful thoughts, images, feelings, and physical sensations are. It may be necessary to stop the narrative at this point and introduce a follow-up session, to decide on how to proceed. In such cases, it may be advisable to postpone the next session until the patient is more stable. In the case of patients with a diagnosis of a borderline personality disorder developing a dissociative state, therapists should be familiar with the use of grounding strategies. These include forced focusing on environmental stimuli or using grounding words, imagery, or objects to help the patient to focus on the here and now (for details, see Baker, Hunter, Lawrence, & David, 2007). Many of these patients have learned specific skills against dissociation, and even when they are in a dissociative state, it may be useful for the therapist to elicit their effective personal strategies. In cases of severe dissociation, it is recommended to terminate the narrative interview and to adapt ASSIP according to the capacities of the patient (e.g., skip the video playback).

Video Playback

As watching the whole video-recorded narrative interview usually takes far too long for the time available in Session 2, it has proven to be helpful for the therapist to decide on the relevant sequence(s) after the first session. The relevant sequences are those with a focus on the circumstances leading to the suicide action. The time span may vary enormously, ranging from weeks (e.g., with developing depressive symptoms) to minutes (in the case of a sudden impulse). In any case the focus should include the triggering event or experience.

It may happen that a patient refuses to watch the video. In this case, we recommend that the patient turns the chair away from the screen, merely listening to the recorded interview. In our experience, the refusal to watch the recorded interview should be seen as a sign of increased suicide risk.

If in the narrative interview, patients showed no or little insight into the suicidal mechanism, the video playback provides an opportunity to prompt for more detailed suicidal cognitions. The therapist may provide his or her own impression from watching the video-recorded interview that the patient seems to find it difficult to talk about the suicidal crisis, thus inviting the patient to help the therapist to understand and empathize with the patient. Generally, most patients find it easier to talk about thought patterns related to the suicidal crisis than about emotions. The therapist may also ask how the notion of suicide as an option in life got into the patient's mind.

Written Summary

It is advisable to write a first draft of the summary right after the first session, and to revise it after the video playback. The focus of the summary should be on the individual biographical vulnerability (life career issues in action theoretical terms) and on the related trigger(s) for the suicidal crisis. When formulating the logic of the suicidal mechanism, the implicit question should be: What kind of future situation could trigger another suicidal crisis?

Vulnerabilities are best formulated in terms of needs. For instance, rejection sensitivity may be expressed as the need to be accepted and respected, separation anxiety as the need to feel secure in a relationship, the fear of failing as the need to meet one's own high expectations, etc. Discrepancies between the ideal self and reality are frequent in suicidal patients.

It is important that the therapist can fully understand the inherent logic in the patient's suicidal development. It may be helpful to adopt a "not understanding" stance, thus getting the patient into the position of having to help the interviewer understand. For example, Mrs. C., a married woman with one child, said that the night before the suicide attempt, she had an argument with her husband and teenage daughter about the daughter going to a party, and she felt devalued by her husband. This is how she explained her suicide attempt that took place the next afternoon. When the interviewer said he didn't quite understand why the suicide attempt happened that afternoon, Mrs. C. came up with a further important detail: She had in the past had problems with alcohol, and at lunch, when the same conflict came up again, father and daughter looked at each other, saying, "Mother has been drinking again, this is why she is being difficult." This was the last straw for the patient – not being respected as a concerned mother but instead being devalued because of her past alcohol problem.

If relevant, the summary must also include mental health problems (e.g., depression as a precipitating factor, the role of antidepressant medication, etc.).

To speed up the process of developing a joint case formulation, the draft text may be sent to patients prior to the next appointment so that they can revise it and bring it back to the next session.

Hope Leporello
It has proven to be helpful to send patients an electronic version of the leporello so that, if necessary, they may revise it in the future. Some patients like to make it more personal by adding a personal picture.

General Remarks
Many patients have a history of serious mental problems that require a long-term therapy. It is important for the ASSIP therapist not to let himself/herself be carried away by therapeutic enthusiasm, but to stay focused on the suicidality issue and in particular the formulation of the suicidal mechanism, the warning signs, and the safety strategies.

Length of the Sessions
In our experience, the time for sessions should not exceed 90 min. This means that with some patients, the therapist has to structure the session and to guide patients back to the relevant issues. In the narrative interviews, most patients are able to tell their story within 30 to 60 min.

3.10   Future Prospects

ASSIP is a dynamic therapy concept that is open for further developments. From the beginning, the ASSIP protocol has been revised and further developed. The authors hope that just as they have revised and improved their interventions, new elements and improvements will be brought by the new users and their experiences. The first edition of the manual was finished as the follow-up evaluation of ASSIP was still under way. The authors decided not to wait for the completion of the assessment to publish the German version of the manual, as another 1 to 2 years would have gone by before the manual could have been published, owing to the time span required to include 120 patients and to follow each of them up over 2 years. Readers will be able to access the main results of the randomized controlled study on the website (http://www.assip.ch) as soon as they are published (expected to be in the course of 2015).

References

Adler, H. M. (1997). The history of the present illness as treatment: Who's listening, and why does it matter? *The Journal of the American Board of Family Practice, 10*, 28–35.

Ainsworth, M. S. (1989). Attachments beyond infancy. *American Psychologist, 44*, 709–716. http://doi.org/10.1037/0003-066X.44.4.709

Ajdacic-Gross, V., Killias, M., Hepp, U., Gadola, E., Bopp, M., Lauber, C., . . . Rössler, W. (2006). Changing times: A longitudinal analysis of international firearm suicide data. *American Journal of Public Health, 96*, 1752–1755. http://doi.org/10.2105/AJPH.2005.075812

Aleman, A., & Denys, D. (2014). Mental health: A road map for suicide research and prevention. *Nature, 509*, 421–423. http://doi.org/10.1038/509421a

Alexander, L. B., & Luborsky, L. (1986). The Penn Helping Alliance Scales. In L. S. Greenberg & W. M. Pinsoff (Eds.), *The psychotherapeutic process: A research handbook* (pp. 325–366). New York, NY: Guilford Press.

Allen, J. (2011). Mentalizing suicidal states. In K. Michel & D. A. Jobes (Eds.), *Building a therapeutic alliance with the suicidal patient* (pp. 81–91). Washington, DC: American Psychological Association, APA Books.

Angst, J., Angst, F., Gerber-Werder, R., & Gamma, A. (2005). Suicide in 406 mood-disorder patients with and without long-term medication: A 40 to 44 years' follow-up. *Archives of Suicide Research, 9*, 279–300. http://doi.org/10.1080/13811110590929488

Arango, V., Underwood, M. D., Boldrini, M., Tamir, H., Kassir, S. A., Hsiung, S., . . . Mann, J. J. (2001). Serotonin 1A receptors, serotonin transporter binding and serotonin transporter mRNA expression in the brainstem of depressed suicide victims. *Neuropsychopharmacology, 25*, 892–903. http://doi.org/10.1016/S0893-133X(01)00310-4

Arango, V., Underwood, M. D., Gubbi, A. V., & Mann, J. J. (1995). Localized alterations in pre- and post-synaptic serotonin binding sites in the ventrolateral prefrontal cortex of suicide victims. *Brain Research, 688*(1–2), 121–133. http://doi.org/10.1016/0006-8993(95)00523-S

Arensman, E., Townsend, E., Hawton, K., Bremner, S., Feldman, E., Goldney, R., . . . Traskman-Bendz, L. (2001). Psychosocial and pharmacological treatment of patients following deliberate self-harm: The methodological issues involved in evaluating effectiveness. *Suicide and Life-Threatening Behavior, 31*, 169–180. http://doi.org/10.1521/suli.31.2.169.21516

Asberg, M. (1997). Neurotransmitters and suicidal behavior. *Annals of the New York Academy of Sciences, 836*, 158–181. http://doi.org/10.1111/j.1749-6632.1997.tb52359.x

Baker, D., Hunter, E., Lawrence, E., & David, A. (2007). *Overcoming depersonalization and feelings of unreality: A self-help guide to using cognitive behavioral techniques*. London, UK: Robinson.

Baldessarini, R. J., & Tondo, L. (2001). Long-term lithium for bipolar disorder. *American Journal of Psychiatry, 158*, 1740–1740. http://doi.org/10.1176/appi.ajp.158.10.1740

Bandura, A., & Walters, R. H. (1963). *Social learning and personality development*. New York, NY: Holt, Rinehart & Winston.

Barraclough, B., Bunch, J., Nelson, B., & Sainsbury, P. (1974). A hundred cases of suicide: clinical aspects. *British Journal of Psychiatry, 125*, 355–373. http://doi.org/10.1192/bjp.125.4.355

Bateman, A., & Fonagy, P. (2001). Treatment of borderline personality disorder with psychoanalytically oriented partial hospitalization: An 18-month follow-up. *American Journal of Psychiatry, 158*, 36–42. http://doi.org/10.1176/appi.ajp.158.1.36

Bateman, A., & Fonagy, P. (2008). 8-year follow-up of patients treated for borderline personality disorder: Mentalization-based treatment versus treatment as usual. *American Journal of Psychiatry, 165*, 631–638. http://doi.org/10.1176/appi.ajp.2007.07040636

Bateman, A. W., & Fonagy, P. (2004). Mentalization-based treatment of BPD. *Journal of Personality Disorders, 18*, 36–51. http://doi.org/10.1521/pedi.18.1.36.32772

Baumeister, R. F. (1990). Suicide as escape from self. *Psychological Review, 97*, 90–113. http://doi.org/10.1037/0033-295X.97.1.90

Baumeister, R. F., & Heatherton, T. F. (1996). Self-regulation failure: An overview. *Psychological Inquiry, 7*, 1–15. http://doi.org/10.1207/s15327965pli0701_1

Beautrais, A. L. (2000). Risk factors for suicide and attempted suicide among young people. *Australian and New Zealand Journal of Psychiatry, 34*, 420–436. http://doi.org/10.1080/j.1440-1614.2000.00691.x

Beautrais, A. L. (2001). Effectiveness of barriers at suicide jumping sites: A case study. *Australasian Psychiatry, 35*, 557–562.

Beautrais, A. L. (2004). Further suicidal behavior among medically serious suicide attempters. *Suicide and Life-Threatening Behavior, 34*, 1–11. http://doi.org/10.1521/suli.34.1.1.27772

Beautrais, A. L. (2007). Suicide by jumping. *Crisis, 28*, 58–63.

Beautrais, A. L., Fergusson, D. M., & Horwood, L. J. (2006). Firearms legislation and reductions in firearm-related suicide deaths in New Zealand. *Australian and New Zealand Journal of Psychiatry, 40*, 253–259. http://doi.org/10.1080/j.1440-1614.2006.01782.x

Beautrais, A. L., Gibb, S. J., Faulkner, A., Fergusson, D. M., & Mulder, R. T. (2010). Postcard intervention for repeat self-harm: Randomised controlled trial. *British Journal of Psychiatry, 197*, 55–60. http://doi.org/10.1192/bjp.bp.109.075754

Beautrais, A. L., Gibb, S. J., Fergusson, D. M., Horwood, L. J., & Larkin, G. L. (2009). Removing bridge barriers stimulates suicides: An unfortunate natural experiment. *The Australian and New Zealand Journal of Psychiatry, 43*, 495–497. http://doi.org/10.1080/00048670902873714

Beck, A. (1976). *Cognitive therapy and the emotional disorders*. New York, NY: New American Library.

Beck, A. T. (1996). Beyond belief: A theory of modes, personality, and psychopathology. In P. Salkovskis (Ed.), *Frontiers of cognitive therapy* (pp. 1–25). New York, NY: Guilford Press.

Beck, A. T., Rush, A. J., Shaw, B. F., & Emery, G. (1979). *Cognitive therapy of depression*. New York, NY: Guilford Press.

Bell, D. (2008). Who is killing what or whom? Some notes on the internal phenomenology of suicide. In S. Briggs, A. Lemma, & W. Crouch (Eds.), *Relating to self-harm and suicide: Psychoanalytic perspectives on theory, practice and prevention* (pp. 38–45). London, UK: Routledge.

Bennewith, O., Evans, J., Donovan, J., Paramasivan, S., Owen-Smith, A., Hollingworth, W., . . . Gunnell, D. (2014). A contact-based intervention for people recently discharged from inpatient psychiatric care: A pilot study. *Archives of Suicide Research, 18*, 131–143. http://doi.org/10.1080/13811118.2013.838196

Bertolote, J. M., & Fleischmann, A. (2002). Suicide and psychiatric diagnosis: A worldwide perspective. *World Psychiatry, 1*, 181–185.

Bostwick, J. M. (2011). Pharmacotherapy and therapeutic alliance in the treatment of suicidality. In K. Michel & D. A. Jobes (Eds.), *Building a therapeutic alliance with the suicidal patient* (pp. 353–375). Washington, DC: American Psychological Association.

Bostwick, J. M., & Pankratz, V. S. (2000). Affective disorders and suicide risk: A reexamination. *American Journal of Psychiatry, 157*, 1925–1932. http://doi.org/10.1176/appi.ajp.157.12.1925

Bowlby, J. (1977a). The making and breaking of affectional bonds: Part I: Aetiology and psychopathology in the light of attachment theory. *British Journal of Psychiatry, 130*(4), 201–210.

Bowlby, J. (1977b). The making and breaking of affectional bonds. Part II. Some principles of psychotherapy. *British Journal of Psychiatry, 130*(5), 421–431.

Bowlby, J. (1980). *Attachment and loss. Vol. 3: Sadness and depression*. New York, NY: Basic Books.

Bowlby, J. (1988). *A secure base: Clinical applications of attachment theory*. London, UK: Routledge.

Bremner, J. D., Narayan, M., Staib, L. H., Southwick, S. M., McGlashan, T., & Charney, D. S. (1999). Neural correlates of memories of childhood sexual abuse in women with and without posttraumatic stress disorder. *American Journal of Psychiatry, 156*, 1787–1795.

Brent, D. A., Bridge, J., Johnson, B. A., & Connolly, J. (1996). Suicidal behavior runs in families. A controlled family study of adolescent suicide victims. *Archives of General Psychiatry, 53*, 1145–1152. http://doi.org/10.1001/archpsyc.1996.01830120085015

Brent, D. A., Johnson, B. A., Perper, J., Connolly, J., Bridge, J., Bartle, S., & Rather, C. (1994). Personality disorder, personality traits, impulsive violence, and completed suicide in adolescents. *Journal of the American Academy of Child & Adolescent Psychiatry, 33*, 1080–1086. http://doi.org/10.1097/00004583-199410000-00003

Bronisch, T. (2008). Suizidalität [Suicidality]. In J.-H. Möller, G. Laux, & H.-P. Krapfhammer (Eds.), *Psychiatrie und psychotherapie* (pp. 2283–2308). Berlin, Germany: Springer.

Bronisch, T., & Wolfersdorf, M. (2012). Definition von Suizidalität: Wie grenzen wir suizidales und nicht-suizidales Verhalten ab? [Definition of suicidality: How do we separate suicidal from nonsuicidal behavior?] *Suizidprophylaxe, 39*, 41–50.

Brown, G. K., & Jager-Hyman, S. (2014). Evidence-based psychotherapies for suicide prevention: Future directions. *American Journal of Preventive Medicine, 47*, S186–S194. http://doi.org/10.1016/j.amepre.2014.06.008

Brown, G. K., Ten Have, T., Henriques, G. R., Xie, S. X., Hollander, J. E., & Beck, A. T. (2005). Cognitive therapy for the prevention of suicide attempts: A randomized controlled trial. *JAMA, 294*, 563–570. http://doi.org/10.1001/jama.294.5.563

Brown, G. K., Wenzel, A., & Rudd, M. D. (2011). Engaging the suicidal patient in cognitive therapy. In K. Michel & D. A. Jobes (Eds.), *Building a therapeutic alliance with the suicidal patient* (pp. 273–291). Washington, DC: American Psychological Association.

Bruffaerts, R., Demyttenaere, K., Borges, G., Haro, J. M., Chiu, W. T., Hwang, I., . . . Nock, M. K. (2010). Childhood adversities as risk factors for onset and persistence of suicidal behaviour. *British Journal of Psychiatry, 197*, 20–27. http://doi.org/10.1192/bjp.bp.109.074716

Buss, A. R. (1978). Causes and reasons in attribution theory: A conceptual critique. *Journal of Personality and Social Psychology, 36*, 1311–1321. http://doi.org/10.1037/0022-3514.36.11.1311

Cannon, W. B. (1929). *Bodily changes in pain hunger fear and rage*. New York, NY: Appleton-Century-Crofts.

Carter, C. S., Botvinick, M. M., & Cohen, J. D. (1999). The contribution of the anterior cingulate cortex to executive processes in cognition. *Reviews in the Neurosciences, 10*, 49–57. http://doi.org/10.1515/REVNEURO.1999.10.1.49

Carter, G. L., Clover, K., Whyte, I. M., Dawson, A. H., & D'Este, C. (2005). Postcards from the EDge project: Randomised controlled trial of an intervention using postcards to reduce repetition of hospital treated deliberate self poisoning. *BMJ, 331*, 805–807. http://doi.org/10.1136/bmj.38579.455266.E0

Carter, G. L., Clover, K., Whyte, I. M., Dawson, A. H., & D'Este, C. (2013). Postcards from the EDge: 5-year outcomes of a randomised controlled trial for hospital-treated self-poisoning. *British Journal of Psychiatry, 202*, 372–380. http://doi.org/10.1192/bjp.bp.112.112664

Carver, C. S., & Scheier, M. (1990). Principles of self-regulation: Action and emotion. In E. T. Higgins & R. M. Sorrentino (Eds.), *Handbook of motivation and cognition: Foundations of social behavior* (Vol. 2, pp. 3–52). New York, NY: Guilford Press.

Caspi, A., Sugden, K., Moffitt, T. E., Taylor, A., Craig, I. W., Harrington, H., . . . Poulton, R. (2003). Influence of life stress on depression: Moderation by a polymorphism in the 5-HTT gene. *Science, 301*, 386–389. http://doi.org/10.1126/science.1083968

Chan, K. P., Yip, P. S., Au, J., & Lee, D. T. (2005). Charcoal-burning suicide in post-transition Hong Kong. *British Journal of Psychiatry, 186*, 67–73. http://doi.org/10.1192/bjp.186.1.67

Chesin, M., & Stanley, B. (2013). Risk assessment and psychosocial interventions for suicidal patients. *Bipolar Disorders, 15*, 584–593. http://doi.org/10.1111/bdi.12092

Cipriani, A., Pretty, H., Hawton, K., & Geddes, J. R. (2005). Lithium in the prevention of suicidal behavior and all-cause mortality in patients with mood disorders: A systematic review of randomized trials. *American Journal of Psychiatry, 162*, 1805–1819. http://doi.org/10.1176/appi.ajp.162.10.1805

Clayton, P. (1983). Epidemiologic and risk factors in suicide. In L. Greenspoon (Ed.), *Psychiatry update* (pp. 428–434). Washington, DC: American Psychiatric Press.

Comer, R. J., & Sartory, G. (1995). *Klinische Psychologie* [Clinical psychology]. Heidelberg, Germany: Spektrum.

Conwell, Y., Duberstein, P. R., Cox, C., Herrmann, J. H., Forbes, N. T., & Caine, E. D. (1996). Relationships of age and axis I diagnoses in victims of completed suicide: A psychological autopsy study. *American Journal of Psychiatry, 153*, 1001–1008. http://doi.org/10.1176/ajp.153.8.1001

Coryell, W., & Schlesser, M. (2001). The dexamethasone suppression test and suicide prediction. *American Journal of Psychiatry, 158*, 748–753. http://doi.org/10.1176/appi.ajp.158.5.748

Cotgrove, A., Zirinsky, L., Black, D., & Weston, D. (1995). Secondary prevention of attempted suicide in adolescence. *Journal of Adolescence, 18*, 569–577. http://doi.org/10.1006/jado.1995.1039

Cox, G. R., Owens, C., Robinson, J., Nicholas, A., Lockley, A., Williamson, M., . . . Pirkis, J. (2013). Interventions to reduce suicides at suicide hotspots: A systematic review. *BMC Public Health, 13*, 214. http://doi.org/10.1186/1471-2458-13-214

Davidson, R. J., Kabat-Zinn, J., Schumacher, J., Rosenkranz, M., Muller, D., Santorelli, S. F., . . . Sheridan, J. F. (2003). Alterations in brain and immune function produced by mindfulness meditation. *Psychosomatic Medicine, 65*, 564–570. http://doi.org/10.1097/01.PSY.0000077505.67574.E3

De Leo, D. (2002). Why are we not getting any closer to preventing suicide? *British Journal of Psychiatry, 181*, 372–374. http://doi.org/10.1192/bjp.181.5.372

De Leo, D., Buono, M. D., & Dwyer, J. (2002). Suicide among the elderly: The long-term impact of a telephone support and assessment intervention in northern Italy. *British Journal of Psychiatry, 181*, 226–229. http://doi.org/10.1192/bjp.181.3.226

Department of Health and Human Services. (2012). *2012 National Strategy for Suicide Prevention: Goals and objectives for action.* Washington, DC: Author. Retrieved from http://www.actionallianceforsuicideprevention.org/NSSP

Dörner, K. (1993). Schnittpunkt des Rechts zu leben und des Rechts zu sterben [Crossroads of the right to live and the right to die]. In Th. Giernalczyk & E. Frick (Eds.), *Suizidalität: Deutungsmuster und Praxisansätze* (pp. 1–10). Regensburg, Germany: Roderer.

Dumais, A., Lesage, A. D., Alda, M., Rouleau, G., Dumont, M., Chawky, N., . . . Turecki, G. (2005). Risk factors for suicide completion in major depression: A case-control study of impulsive and aggressive behaviors in men. *American Journal of Psychiatry, 162*, 2116–2124. http://doi.org/10.1176/appi.ajp.162.11.2116

Durkheim, E. (1897, German trans. 1973). *Le suicide: Étude de sociologie* [Suicide: A study in sociology] (S. u. H. Herkommer, German Trans.). Neuwied/Berlin: Luchterhand. (Original work published Paris: Félix Alcan.

Epstein, S., Pacini, R., Denes-Raj, V., & Heier, H. (1996). Individual differences in intuitive–experiential and analytical–rational thinking styles. *Journal of Personality and Social Psychology, 71*, 390–405. http://doi.org/10.1037/0022-3514.71.2.390

Etzersdorfer, E., & Sonneck, G. (1998). Preventing suicide by influencing mass-media reporting: The Viennese experience 1980–1996. *Archives of Suicide Research, 4*, 67–74. http://doi.org/10.1023/A:1009691903261

Fergusson, D., Doucette, S., Glass, K. C., Shapiro, S., Healy, D., Hebert, P., & Hutton, B. (2005). Association between suicide attempts and selective serotonin reuptake inhibitors: Systematic review of randomised controlled trials. *BMJ, 330*, 396–399. http://doi.org/10.1136/bmj.330.7488.396

Feuerlein, W. (1971). Selbstmordversuch oder parasuizidale Handlung [Attempted suicide or parasuicidal behavior]. *Nervenarzt, 42*, 109–114.

Fonagy, P., Gergely, G., Jurist, E. L., & Target, M. (2004). *Affect regulation, mentalization and the development of the self.* London, UK: Karnac Books.

Freeling, P., Rao, B. M., Paykel, E. S., Sireling, L. I., & Burton, R. H. (1985). Unrecognised depression in general practice. *BMJ (Clinical Research Ed.), 290*, 1880–1883.

Freud, S. (1917). *Mourning and melancholia. The standard edition of the complete psychological works of Sigmund Freud, Volume XIV (1914–1916): On the history of the psycho-analytic movement, papers on metapsychology and other works* (Vol. 14). London, UK: Hogarth Press.

Gaston, L., Thompson, L., Gallagher, D., Cournoyer, L., & Gagnon, R. (1998). Alliance, technique, and their interactions in predicting outcome of behavioural, cognitive, and brief dynamic therapy. *Psychotherapy Research, 8*, 190–209. http://doi.org/10.1080/10503309812331332307

Gibbons, R. D., Brown, C. H., Hur, K., Marcus, S. M., Bhaumik, D. K., Erkens, J. A., . . . Mann, J. J. (2007). Early evidence on the effects of regulators' suicidality warnings on SSRI prescriptions and suicide in children and adolescents. *American Journal of Psychiatry, 164*, 1356–1363. http://doi.org/10.1176/appi.ajp.2007.07030454

Gibb, S. J., Beautrais, A. L., & Fergusson, D. M. (2005). Mortality and further suicidal behaviour after an index suicide attempt: A 10-year study. *Australian and New Zealand Journal of Psychiatry, 39*(1–2), 95–100. http://doi.org/10.1080/j.1440-1614.2005.01514.x

Goldsmith, S. K., Pellmar, T. C., Kleinman, A. M., & Bunney, W. E. (2002). *Reducing suicide: A national imperative.* Washington, DC: National Academies Press.

Goodwin, F. K., & Jamison, K. R. (1990). *Manic-depressive illness.* New York, NY: Oxford University Press.

Grawe, K. (2004). *Psychological therapy.* Seattle, WA: Hogrefe.

Grimholt, T. K., Bjornaas, M. A., Jacobsen, D., Dieserud, G., & Ekeberg, O. (2012). Treatment received, satisfaction with health care services, and psychiatric symptoms 3 months after hospitalization for self-poisoning. *Annals of General Psychiatry, 11*, 10.

Guthrie, E., Kapur, N., Mackway-Jones, K., Chew-Graham, C., Moorey, J., Mendel, E., . . . Tomenson, B. (2001). Randomised controlled trial of brief psychological intervention after deliberate self poisoning. *BMJ, 323*, 135–138. http://doi.org/10.1136/bmj.323.7305.135

Gysin-Maillart, A., Soravia, L., Gemperli, A., & Michel, K. (2015). *Effects of therapeutic alliance on suicidal ideation in ASSIP, a brief therapy for attempted suicide.* Manuscript submitted for publication.

Harris, E. C., & Barraclough, B. (1997). Suicide as an outcome for mental disorders: A meta-analysis. *British Journal of Psychiatry, 170*, 205–228. http://doi.org/10.1192/bjp.170.3.205

Hartley, D. E., & Strupp, H. H. (1983). The therapeutic alliance: Its relationship to outcome in brief psychotherapy. In J. Masling & N. J. Hillsdale (Eds.), *Empirical studies of psychoanalytic theories* (Vol. 1, pp. 1–37). Hillsdale, NJ: Erlbaum.

Haw, C., Bergen, H., Casey, D., & Hawton, K. (2007). Repetition of deliberate self-harm: A study of the characteristics and subsequent deaths in patients presenting to a general hospital according to extent of repetition. *Suicide and Life-Threatening Behavior, 37*, 379–396. http://doi.org/10.1521/suli.2007.37.4.379

Hawton, K., Arensman, E., Wasserman, D., Hulten, A., Bille-Brahe, U., Bjerke, T., . . . Temesvary, B. (1998). Relation between attempted suicide and suicide rates among young people in Europe. *Journal of Epidemiology and Community Health, 52*, 191–194. http://doi.org/10.1136/jech.52.3.191

Hawton, K., Bergen, H., Simkin, S., Brock, A., Griffiths, C., Romeri, E., . . . Gunnell, D. (2009). Effect of withdrawal of co-proxamol on prescribing and deaths from drug poisoning in England and Wales: Time series analysis. *BMJ, 338*, 2270. http://doi.org/10.1136/bmj.b2270

Hawton, K., & Blackstock, E. (1976). General practice aspects of self-poisoning and self-injury. *Psychological Medicine, 6*, 571–575. http://doi.org/10.1017/S0033291700018195

Hawton, K., Simkin, S., Deeks, J., Cooper, J., Johnston, A., Waters, K., . . . Hudson, M. (2004). UK legislation on analgesic packs: Before and after study of long term effect on poisonings. *BMJ, 329*, 1076–1079. http://doi.org/10.1136/bmj.38253.572581.7C

Hawton, K., Townsend, E., Deeks, J., Appleby, L., Gunnell, D., Bennewith, O., & Cooper, J. (2001). Effects of legislation restricting pack sizes of paracetamol and salicylate on self poisoning in the United Kingdom: Before and after study. *BMJ, 322*, 1203–1207.

Hawton, K., Zahl, D., & Weatherall, R. (2003). Suicide following deliberate self-harm: Long-term follow-up of patients who presented to a general hospital. *British Journal of Psychiatry, 182*, 537–542. http://doi.org/10.1192/bjp.182.6.537

Hegerl, U., Althaus, D., Schmidtke, A., & Niklewski, G. (2006). The alliance against depression: 2-year evaluation of a community-based intervention to reduce suicidality. *Psychological Medicine, 36*, 1225–1233. http://doi.org/10.1017/S003329170600780X

Hegerl, U., Wittmann, M., Arensman, E., Van Audenhove, C., Bouleau, J.-H., Van der Feltz-Cornelis, C., . . . Maxwell, M. (2008). The 'European Alliance Against Depression (EAAD)': A multifaceted, community-based action programme against depression and suicidality. *World Journal of Biological Psychiatry, 9*, 51–58.

Heider, F. (1958). *The psychology of interpersonal relations.* New York, NY: Wiley. http://doi.org/10.1037/10628-000

Heikkinen, M. E., Isometsä, E., Marttunen, M. J., & Aro, H. M. (1995). Social factors in suicide. *British Journal of Psychiatry, 167*, 747–753. http://doi.org/10.1192/bjp.167.6.747

Heim, C., Young, L. J., Newport, D. J., Mletzko, T., Miller, A. H., & Nemeroff, C. B. (2009). Lower CSF oxytocin concentrations in women with a history of childhood abuse. *Molecular Psychiatry, 14*, 954–958. http://doi.org/10.1038/mp.2008.112

Henseler, H. (1974). *Narzisstische Krisen* [Narcissist crises]. Hamburg, Germany: Rowohlt.

Hepp, U., Wittmann, L., Schnyder, U., & Michel, K. (2004). Psychological and psychosocial interventions after attempted suicide: An overview of treatment studies. *Crisis, 25*, 108–117.

Hermans, H. J. M., & Hermans-Jansen, E. (1995). *Self-narratives: The construction of meaning in psychotherapy.* New York, NY: Guilford Press.

Hjelmeland, H., & Hawton, K. (2004). Intentional aspects of non-fatal suicidal behaviour. In D. De Leo, U. Bille-Brahe, & A. Kerkhof (Eds.), *Attempted suicide: A handbook of treatment, theory, and recent findings* (pp. 67–68). Göttingen, Germany: Hogrefe & Huber.

Holmes, J. (2001). *The search for the secure base: Attachment theory and psychotherapy.* Hove, UK: Brunner Routledge.

Holmes, J. (2006). Mentalizing from a psychoanalytic perspective: What's new. In J. Allen & P. Fonagy (Eds.), *Handbook of mentalisation-based treatment* (pp. 31–49). Chichester, UK: Wiley.

Holmes, J. (2011). Attachment theory and the suicidal patient. In K. Michel & D. A. Jobes (Eds.), *Building a therapeutic alliance with the suicidal patient* (pp. 149–168). Washington, DC: American Psychological Association.

Horvath, A. O., Gaston, L., & Luborsky, L. (1993). The therapeutic alliance and its measures. In L. L. N. Miller, J. Barber, & J. P. Docherty (Eds.), *Psychodynamic treatment research* (pp. 247–273) New York: Basic Books.

Horvath, A. O., & Symonds, B. D. (1991). Relation between working alliance and outcome in psychotherapy: A meta-analysis. *Journal of Counseling Psychology, 38*, 139–149. http://doi.org/10.1037/0022-0167.38.2.139

Hoyert, D. L., Kung, H.-C., & Smith, B. L. (2005). Deaths: Preliminary data for 2003. *National Vital Statistics Reports, 53*, 1–48.

Isacsson, G. (2000). Suicide prevention: A medical breakthrough? *Acta Psychiatrica Scandinavica, 102*, 113–117. http://doi.org/10.1034/j.1600-0447.2000.102002113.x

Isacsson, G., Holmgren, P., Wasserman, D., & Bergman, U. (1994). Use of antidepressants among people committing suicide in Sweden. *BMJ, 308*, 506–509. http://doi.org/10.1136/bmj.308.6927.506

Isometsä, E. T., Henriksson, M., Aro, H. M., & Lönnqvist, J. K. (1994). Suicide in bipolar disorder in Finland. *American Journal of Psychiatry, 151*, 1020–1024. http://doi.org/10.1176/ajp.151.7.1020

Isometsä, E., Henriksson, M., Heikkinen, M., Aro, H., & Lonnqvist, J. (1994). Suicide and the use of antidepressants: Drug treatment of depression is inadequate. *BMJ, 308*, 915. http://doi.org/10.1136/bmj.308.6933.915

Isometsä, E., Henriksson, M., Marttunen, M., Heikkinen, M., Aro, H., Kuoppasalmi, K., & Lonnqvist, J. (1995). Mental disorders in young and middle aged men who commit suicide. *BMJ, 310*, 1366–1367. http://doi.org/10.1136/bmj.310.6991.1366

Isometsä, E. T., Heikkinen, M. E., Marttunen, M. J., Henriksson, M. M., Aro, H. M., & Lönnqvist, J. K. (1995). The last appointment before suicide: Is suicide intent communicated? *American Journal of Psychiatry, 152*, 919–922. http://doi.org/10.1176/ajp.152.6.919

Jenkins, G. R., Hale, R., Papanastassiou, M., Crawford, M. J., & Tyrer, P. (2002). Suicide rate 22 years after parasuicide: Cohort study. *BMJ, 325*, 1155. http://doi.org/10.1136/bmj.325.7373.1155

Jobes, D. A. (1995). The challenge and the promise of clinical suicidology. *Suicide and Life-Threatening Behavior, 25*, 437–449

Jobes, D. A. (2000). Collaborating to prevent suicide: A clinical-research perspective. *Suicide and Life-Threatening Behavior, 30*, 8–17.

Jobes, D. A. (2006). *Managing suicidal risk: A collaborative approach.* New York, NY: Guilford Press.

Jobes, D. A. (2011). Suicidal patients, the therapeutic alliance, and the collaborative assessment and management of suicidality. In K. Michel & D. A. Jobes (Eds.), *Building a therapeutic alliance with the suicidal patient* (pp. 205–229). Washington, DC: American Psychological Association.

Jobes, D. A. (2012). The collaborative assessment and management of suicidality (CAMS): An evolving evidence-based clinical approach to suicidal risk. *Suicide and Life-Threatening Behavior, 42*, 640–653.

Johannessen, H. A., Dieserud, G., De Leo, D., Claussen, B., & Zahl, P.-H. (2011). Chain of care for patients who have attempted suicide: A follow-up study from Bærum, Norway. *BMC public health, 11*, 81. http://doi.org/10.1186/1471-2458-11-81

Joiner, T. E. (2005). *Why people die by suicide.* Cambridge, MA: Harvard University Press.

Jollant, F., Bellivier, F., Leboyer, M., Astruc, B., Torres, S., Verdier, R., . . . Courtet, P. (2005). Impaired decision making in suicide attempters. *American Journal of Psychiatry, 162*, 304–310. http://doi.org/10.1176/appi.ajp.162.2.304

Kagan, N., Krathwohl, D. R., & Miller, R. (1963). Stimulated recall in therapy using video tape: A case study. *Journal of Counseling Psychology, 10*, 237–243. http://doi.org/10.1037/h0045497

Kahneman, D. (2011). *Thinking fast and slow.* New York, NY: Farrar, Strauss and Giroux.

Kapur, N., Gunnell, D., Hawton, K., Nadeem, S., Khalil, S., Longson, D., . . . Cooper, J. (2013). Messages from Manchester: Pilot randomised controlled trial following self-harm. *British Journal of Psychiatry, 203*, 73–74. http://doi.org/10.1192/bjp.bp.113.126425

Kessler, R. C., Berglund, P., Borges, G., Nock, M., & Wang, P. S. (2005). Trends in suicide ideation, plans, gestures, and attempts in the United States, 1990–1992 to 2001–2003. *JAMA, 293*, 2487–2495. http://doi.org/10.1001/jama.293.20.2487

Kessler, R. C., Borges, G., & Walters, E. E. (1999). Prevalence of and risk factors for lifetime suicide attempts in the National Comorbidity Survey. *Archives of General Psychiatry, 56*, 617–626. http://doi.org/10.1001/archpsyc.56.7.617

Khan, A., Khan, S., Kolts, R., & Brown, W. A. (2003). Suicide rates in clinical trials of SSRIs, other antidepressants, and placebo: Analysis of FDA reports. *American Journal of Psychiatry, 160*, 790–792. http://doi.org/10.1176/appi.ajp.160.4.790

Kleiman, E. M., & Liu, R. T. (2014). Prospective prediction of suicide in a nationally representative sample: Religious service attendance as a protective factor. *British Journal of Psychiatry, 204*, 262–266. http://doi.org/10.1192/bjp.bp.113.128900

Kohut, H. (1971). *The analysis of the self: A systematic approach to the psychoanalytic treatment of narcissistic personality disorders.* New York, NY: International Universities Press.

Krupnick, J. L., Sotsky, S. M., Simmens, S., Moyer, J., Elkin, I., Watkins, J., & Pilkonis, P. A. (1996). The role of the therapeutic alliance in psychotherapy and pharmacotherapy outcome: Findings in the National Institute of Mental Health Treatment of Depression Collaborative Research Program. *Journal of Consulting and Clinical Psychology, 64*, 532–539. http://doi.org/10.1037/0022-006X.64.3.532

Kurz, A., Möller, H. J., Bürk, F., Torhorst, A., Wächtler, C., & Lauter, H. (1988). Evaluation of two different aftercare strategies of an outpatient aftercare program for suicide attempters in a general hospital. In H. J. Möller, A. Schmidtke, & R. Welz (Eds.), *Current issues in suicidology* (pp. 414–418). Berlin, Germany: Springer.

Labonte, B., & Turecki, G. (2010). The epigenetics of suicide: Explaining the biological effects of early life environmental adversity. *Archives of Suicide Research, 14*, 291–310. http://doi.org/10.1080/13811118.2010.524025

Lanius, R. A., Williamson, P. C., Densmore, M., Boksman, K., Gupta, M. A., Neufeld, R. W., . . . Menon, R. S. (2001). Neural correlates of traumatic memories in posttraumatic stress disorder: A functional MRI investigation. *American Journal of Psychiatry, 158*, 1920–1922. http://doi.org/10.1176/appi.ajp.158.11.1920

Larkin, G. L., & Beautrais, A. L. (2010). Emergency departments are underutilized sites for suicide prevention. *Crisis, 31*, 1–6. http://doi.org/10.1027/0227-5910/a000001

Leenaars, A. (1988). *Suicide notes.* New York, NY: Human Sciences Press.

Lin, E. H., Von Korff, M., & Wagner, E. H. (1989). Identifying suicide potential in primary care. *Journal of General Internal Medicine, 4*, 1–6. http://doi.org/10.1007/BF02596482

Linehan, M. M. (1993a). *Cognitive behavioural therapy of borderline personality disorder.* New York, NY: Guilford Press.

Linehan, M. M. (1993b). *Skills training manual for treating borderline personality disorder.* New York, NY: Guilford Press.

Linehan, M. M. (1997). Validation and psychotherapy. In A. C. Bohart & L. Greenberg (Eds.), *Empathy reconsidered: New directions in psychotherapy* (pp. 353–392). Washington, DC: American Psychological Association.

Linehan, M. M. (2008). Suicide intervention research: A field in desperate need of development. *Suicide and Life-Threatening Behavior, 38*, 483–485. http://doi.org/10.1521/suli.2008.38.5.483

Linehan, M. M., Comtois, K. A., Murray, A. M., Brown, M. Z., Gallop, R. J., Heard, H. L., . . . Lindenboim, N. (2006). Two-year randomized controlled trial and follow-up of dialectical behavior therapy vs therapy by experts for suicidal behaviors and borderline personality disorder. *Archives of General Psychiatry, 63*, 757–766. http://doi.org/10.1001/archpsyc.63.7.757

Linehan, M. M., Goodstein, J. L., Nielsen, S. L., & Chiles, J. A. (1983). Reasons for staying alive when you are thinking of killing yourself: The reasons for living inventory. *Journal of Consulting and Clinical Psychology, 51*, 276–286. http://doi.org/10.1037/0022-006X.51.2.276

Lizardi, D., & Stanley, B. (2010). Treatment engagement: A neglected aspect in the psychiatric care of suicidal patients. *Psychiatric Services, 61*, 1183–1191. http://doi.org/10.1176/appi.ps.61.12.1183

Lopez, A. D., Mathers, C. D., Ezzati, M., Jamison, D. T., & Murray, C. J. (2006). Global and regional burden of disease and risk factors, 2001: Systematic analysis of population health data. *The Lancet, 367*, 1747–1757. http://doi.org/10.1016/S0140-6736(06)68770-9

Luxton, D. D., June, J. D., & Comtois, K. A. (2013). Can postdischarge follow-up contacts prevent suicide and suicidal behavior? A review of the evidence. *Crisis, 34*, 32–41.

Maltsberger, J. T. (1993). Confusions of the body, the self, and others in suicidal states. In A. A. Leenaars (Ed.), *Suicidology: Essays in honor of Edwin S. Shneidman* (pp. 148–171). Northvale, NJ: Jason Aronson.

Maltsberger, J. T. (2004). The descent into suicide. *The International Journal of Psychoanalysis, 85*, 653–668. http://doi.org/10.1516/3C96-URET-TLWX-6LWU

Maltsberger, J. T., & Buie, D. H. (1974). Countertransference hate in the treatment of suicidal patients. *Archives of General Psychiatry, 30*, 625–633. http://doi.org/10.1001/archpsyc.1974.01760110049005

Mann, J. J., Waternaux, C., Haas, G. L., & Malone, K. M. (1999). Toward a clinical model of suicidal behavior in psychiatric patients. *American Journal of Psychiatry, 156*, 181–189.

Maris, R. (1981). *Pathways to suicide: A survey of self-destructive behaviors*. Baltimore, MD: Johns Hopkins University Press.

Maris, R., Berman, A., & Silverman, M. M. (2000). Racial, ethnic, and cultural aspects of suicide. In R. W. Maris, A. L. Berman, & M. M. Silverman (Eds.), *Comprehensive textbook of suicidology* (pp. 182). New York, NY: Guiford Press.

Marzuk, P. M., Tardiff, K., Leon, A. C., Hirsch, C. S., Stajic, M., Hartwell, N., & Portera, L. (1995). Use of prescription psychotropic drugs among suicide victims in New York City. *American Journal of Psychiatry, 152*, 1520–1522. http://doi.org/10.1176/ajp.152.10.1520

Matthews, S., Spadoni, A., Knox, K., Strigo, I., & Simmons, A. (2012). Combat-exposed war veterans at risk for suicide show hyperactivation of prefrontal cortex and anterior cingulate during error processing. *Psychosomatic Medicine, 74*, 471–475. http://doi.org/10.1097/PSY.0b013e31824f888f

McGowan, P. O., Sasaki, A., D'Alessio, A. C., Dymov, S., Labonté, B., Szyf, M., . . . Meaney, M. J. (2009). Epigenetic regulation of the glucocorticoid receptor in human brain associates with childhood abuse. *Nature Neuroscience, 12*, 342–348. http://doi.org/10.1038/nn.2270

McIntosh, J. L., & Drapeau, C. W. (2014). *U.S.A. suicide 2013: Official final data*. Retrieved from http://www.suicidology.org/Portals/14/docs/Resources/FactSheets/2013datapgsv2alt.pdf

Michel, K. (1988). Suicide in young people is different. *Crisis, 9*, 135–145.

Michel, K. (2011). General aspects of therapeutic alliance. In K. Michel & D. A. Jobes (Eds.), *Building a therapeutic alliance with the suicidal patient* (pp. 13–28). Washington, DC: American Psychological Association APA Books.

Michel, K. (2014). Will new insights into neural networks help us improve our models of suicidal behavior? *Crisis, 35*, 215–218.

Michel, K., Dey, P., Stadler, K., & Valach, L. (2004). Therapist sensitivity towards emotional life-career issues and the working alliance with suicide attempters. *Archives of Suicide Research, 8*, 203–213. http://doi.org/10.1080/13811110490436792

Michel, K., Dey, P., & Valach, L. (2001). Suicide as goal-directed action. In K. v. Heeringen (Ed.), *Understanding suicidal behaviour: The Suicidal process approach to research and treatment*. Chichester, UK: Wiley.

Michel, K., Frey, C., Wyss, K., & Valach, L. (2000). An exercise in improving suicide reporting in print media. *Crisis, 21*, 71–79.

Michel, K., & Jobes, D. A. (2011). *Building a therapeutic alliance with the suicidal patient*. Washington, DC: American Psychological Association. http://doi.org/10.1037/12303-000

Michel, K., Maltsberger, J. T., Jobes, D. A., Leenaars, A. A., Orbach, I., Stadler, K., . . . Valach, L. (2002). Discovering the truth in attempted suicide. *American Journal of Psychotherapy, 56*, 424–437.

Michel, K., & Valach, L. (1997). Suicide as goal-directed action. *Archives of Suicide Research, 3*, 213–221. http://doi.org/10.1080/13811119708258273

Michel, K., & Valach, L. (2011). The narrative interview with the suicidal patient. In K. Michel & D. A. Jobes (Eds.), *Building a therapeutic alliance with the suicidal patient* (pp. 63–80). Washington, DC: American Psychological Association.

Michel, K., Valach, L., & Waeber, V. (1994). Understanding deliberate self-harm: The patients' views. *Crisis, 15*, 172–178.

Miller, M., Azrael, D., Hepburn, L., Hemenway, D., & Lippmann, S. J. (2006). The association between changes in household firearm ownership and rates of suicide in the United States, 1981–2002. *Injury Prevention, 12*, 178–182. http://doi.org/10.1136/ip.2005.010850

Morgan, H. G., Jones, E. M., & Owen, J. H. (1993). Secondary prevention of non-fatal deliberate self-harm. The green card study. *British Journal of Psychiatry, 163*, 111–112. http://doi.org/10.1192/bjp.163.1.111

Morthorst, B., Krogh, J., Erlangsen, A., Alberdi, F., & Nordentoft, M. (2012). Effect of assertive outreach after suicide attempt in the AID (assertive intervention for deliberate self harm) trial: Randomised controlled trial. *BMJ, 345*, e4972. http://doi.org/10.1136/bmj.e4972

Motto, J. A., & Bostrom, A. G. (2001). A randomized controlled trial of postcrisis suicide prevention. *Psychiatric Services, 52*, 828–833. http://doi.org/10.1176/appi.ps.52.6.828

Muller-Oerlinghausen, B., Muser-Causemann, B., & Volk, J. (1992). Suicides and parasuicides in a high-risk patient group on and off lithium long-term medication. *Journal of Affective Disorders, 25*, 261–269. http://doi.org/10.1016/0165-0327(92)90084-J

Murphy, G. E. (1975). The physician's responsibility for suicide: Part II: Errors of omission. *Annals of Internal Medicine, 82*, 305–309. http://doi.org/10.7326/0003-4819-82-3-301

National Action Alliance for Suicide Prevention. (2014). *A prioritized research agenda for suicide prevention: An action plan to save lives.* Rockville, MD: National Institute of Mental Health and the Research Prioritization Task Force. Retrieved from http://actionallianceforsuicideprevention.org/task-force/research-prioritization

Nock, M. K., Borges, G., Bromet, E. J., Alonso, J., Angermeyer, M., Beautrais, A., . . . Williams, D. (2008). Cross-national prevalence and risk factors for suicidal ideation, plans and attempts. *British Journal of Psychiatry, 192*, 98–105. http://doi.org/10.1192/bjp.bp.107.040113

Nock, M. K., Hwang, I., Sampson, N. A., & Kessler, R. C. (2010). Mental disorders, comorbidity and suicidal behavior: Results from the National Comorbidity Survey replication. *Molecular Psychiatry, 15*, 868–876. http://doi.org/10.1038/mp.2009.29

OECD. (2013). *OECD health statistics 2013.* Retrieved from http://dx.doi.org/10.1787/health-data-en

Olfson, M., Marcus, S. C., Tedeschi, M., & Wan, G. J. (2006). Continuity of antidepressant treatment for adults with depression in the United States. *American Journal of Psychiatry, 163*, 101–108. http://doi.org/10.1176/appi.ajp.163.1.101

Oquendo, M. A., Kamali, M., Ellis, S. P., Grunebaum, M. F., Malone, K. M., Brodsky, B. S., . . . Mann, J. J. (2002). Adequacy of antidepressant treatment after discharge and the occurrence of suicidal acts in major depression: A prospective study. *American Journal of Psychiatry, 159*, 1746–1751. http://doi.org/10.1176/appi.ajp.159.10.1746

Oquendo, M. A., Placidi, G. P., Malone, K. M., Campbell, C., Keilp, J., Brodsky, B., . . . Mann, J. J. (2003). Positron emission tomography of regional brain metabolic responses to a serotonergic challenge and lethality of suicide attempts in major depression. *Archives of General Psychiatry, 60*, 14–22. http://doi.org/10.1001/archpsyc.60.1.14

Orbach, I. (1994). Dissociation, physical pain, and suicide: A hypothesis. *Suicide and Life-Threatening Behavior, 24*, 68–79.

Orbach, I. (2001). Therapeutic empathy with the suicidal wish: Principles of therapy with suicidal individuals. *American Journal of Psychotherapy, 55*, 166–184.

Orbach, I. (2003). Suicide and the suicidal body. *Suicide and Life-Threatening Behavior, 33*, 1–8. http://doi.org/10.1521/suli.33.1.1.22786

Orbach, I. (2011). Taking an inside view: Stories of pain. In K. Michel & D. A. Jobes (Eds.), *Building a therapeutic alliance with the suicidal patient* (pp. 111–128). Washington, DC: American Psychological Association.

Owens, D., Horrocks, J., & House, A. (2002). Fatal and non-fatal repetition of self-harm: Systematic review. *British Journal of Psychiatry, 181*, 193–199. http://doi.org/10.1192/bjp.181.3.193

Paulus, M. P., Hozack, N., Zauscher, B., McDowell, J. E., Frank, L., Brown, G. G., & Braff, D. L. (2001). Prefrontal, parietal, and temporal cortex networks underlie decision-making in the presence of uncertainty. *Neuroimage, 13*, 91–100. http://doi.org/10.1006/nimg.2000.0667

Phillips, D. P. (1974). The influence of suggestion on suicide: Substantive and theoretical implications of the Werther effect. *American Sociological Review, 39*, 340–354. http://doi.org/10.2307/2094294

Phillips, M. R., Li, X., & Zhang, Y. (2002). Suicide rates in China, 1995–99. *The Lancet, 359*, 835–840. http://doi.org/10.1016/S0140-6736(02)07954-0

Pirkis, J., & Nordentoft, M. (2011). Media influences on suicide and attempted suicide. In R. O'Connor, S. Platt, & J. Gordon (Eds.), *International handbook of suicide prevention: Research, policy and practice* (pp. 531–544). Chichester, UK: Wiley.

Pirkis, J., Spittal, M., Cox, G., Robinson, J., Cheung, Y.-T., & Studdert, D. (2013). The effectiveness of structural interventions at suicide hotspots: A meta-analysis. *International Journal of Epidemiology, 42*, 541–548. http://doi.org/10.1093/ije/dyt021

Placidi, G. P., Oquendo, M. A., Malone, K. M., Huang, Y. Y., Ellis, S. P., & Mann, J. J. (2001). Aggressivity, suicide attempts, and depression: Relationship to cerebrospinal fluid monoamine metabolite levels. *Biological Psychiatry, 50*, 783–791. http://doi.org/10.1016/S0006-3223(01)01170-2

Platt, S. (1984). Unemployment and suicidal behaviour: A review of the literature. *Social Science & Medicine, 19*, 93–115. http://doi.org/10.1016/0277-9536(84)90276-4

Platt, S., Bille-Brahe, U., Kerkhof, A., Schmidtke, A., Bjerke, T., Crepet, P., . . . Michel, K. (1992). Parasuicide in Europe: The WHO/EURO multicentre study on parasuicide: Part I: Introduction and preliminary analysis for 1989. *Acta Psychiatrica Scandinavica, 85*, 97–104.

Platt, S., & Hawton, K. (2000). Suicidal behaviour and the labour market. In K. Hawton & K. van Heeringen (Ed.), *The international handbook of suicide and attempted suicide* (pp. 309–384). Chichester, UK: Wiley.

Pöldinger, W. (1968). *Die Abschätzung der Suizidalität* [Assessment of suicidality]. Bern, Switzerland: Huber.

Reisch, T., & Michel, K. (2005). Securing a suicide hot spot: Effects of a safety net at the Bern Muenster Terrace. *Suicide and Life-Threatening Behavior, 35*, 460–467. http://doi.org/10.1521/suli.2005.35.4.460

Reisch, T., Seifritz, E., Esposito, F., Wiest, R., Valach, L., & Michel, K. (2010). An fMRI study on mental pain and suicidal behavior. *Journal of Affective Disorders, 126*, 321–325. http://doi.org/10.1016/j.jad.2010.03.005

Reisch, T., Steffen, T., Habenstein, A., & Tschacher, W. (2013). Change in suicide rates in Switzerland before and after firearm restriction resulting from the 2003 "Army XXI" reform. *American Journal of Psychiatry, 170*, 977–984. http://doi.org/10.1176/appi.ajp.2013.12091256

Reisch, T., Steffen, T., Maillart, A., & Michel, K. (2010). *Monitoring des suizidalen Verhaltens in der Agglomeration Bern* [Monitoring of suicidal behavior in the Bern agglomeration] [Electronic version]. Retrieved from http://www.bag.admin.ch/themen/medizin/00683/01915/index.html?lang=de

Resick, P. A., & Schnicke, M. (1993). *Cognitive processing therapy for rape victims: A treatment manual* (*Vol. 4*). Newbury Park, CA: Sage.

Rich, C. L., Warstadt, G. M., Nemiroff, R. A., Fowler, R. C., & Young, D. (1991). Suicide, stressors, and the life cycle. *American Journal of Psychiatry, 148*, 524–527.

Ringel, E. (1953). *Der Selbstmord. Abschluß einer krankhaften Entwicklung* [Suicide: Endpoint of a pathologial development]. Düsseldorf: Maudrich.

Rizvi, S. (2011). The therapeutic relationship in dialectical behaviour therapy. In K. Michel & D. A. Jobes (Eds.), *Building a therapeutic alliance with the suicidal patient* (pp. 255–271). Washington, DC: American Psychological Association.

Robins, E., Murphy, G. E., Wilkinson Jr, R. H., Gassner, S., & Kayes, J. (1959). Some clinical considerations in the prevention of suicide based on a study of 134 successful suicides. *American Journal of Public Health and the Nations Health, 49*, 888–899. http://doi.org/10.2105/AJPH.49.7.888

Rogers, J. R., & Soyka, K. M. (2004). "One size fits all": An existential-constructivist perspective on the crisis intervention approach with suicidal individuals. *Journal of Contemporary Psychotherapy, 34*, 7–22. http://doi.org/10.1023/B:JOCP.0000010910.74165.3a

Roy, A., Sarchiapone, M., & Carli, V. (2007). Low resilience in suicide attempters. *Archives of Suicide Research, 11*, 265–269. http://doi.org/10.1080/13811110701403916

Rudd, M. D. (2000). The suicidal mode: A cognitive-behavioral model of suicidality. *Suicide and Life-Threatening Behavior, 30*, 18–33.

Rudd, M. D., Berman, A. L., Joiner, T. E., Jr., Nock, M. K., Silverman, M. M., Mandrusiak, M., . . . Witte, T. (2006). Warning signs for suicide: Theory, research, and clinical applications. *Suicide and Life-Threatening Behavior, 36*, 255–262. http://doi.org/10.1521/suli.2006.36.3.255

Rudd, M. D., & Brown, G. K. (2011). A cognitive theory of suicide: Building hope in treatment and strengthening the therapeutic relationship. In K. Michel & D. A. Jobes (Eds.), *Building a therapeutic alliance with the suicidal patient* (pp. 169–182). Washington, DC: American Psychological Association.

Rudd, M. D., Joiner, T., Brown, G. K., Cukrowicz, K., Jobes, D. A., Silverman, M., & Cordero, L. (2009). Informed consent with suicidal patients: Rethinking risks in (and out of) treatment. *Psychotherapy: Theory, Research, Practice, Training, 46*, 459–468. http://doi.org/10.1037/a0017902

Rudd, M. D., Joiner, T., & Rajab, M. H. (2001). *Treating suicidal behavior: An effective, time-limited approach*. New York, NY: Guilford Press.

Runeson, B. S. (2002). Suicide after parasuicide. *BMJ, 325,* 1125–1126. http://doi.org/10.1136/bmj.325.7373.1125/a

Rutz, W. (2010). Depression und Suizidalität bei Männern in Europa: Ein Problem männlichen psychischen Leidens und männlicher Suizidalität [Male depression and suicidality in Europe: A problem of male mental suffering and male suicidality]. *Journal für Neurologie, Neurochirurgie und Psychiatrie, 11,* 46–52.

Rutz, W., von Knorring, L., Pihlgren, H., Rihmer, Z., & Walinder, J. (1995). Prevention of male suicides: Lessons from Gotland study. *The Lancet, 345,* 524. http://doi.org/10.1016/S0140-6736(95)90622-3

Rutz, W., Walinder, J., Eberhard, G., Holmberg, G., von Knorring, A. L., von Knorring, L., . . . Aberg-Wistedt, A. (1989). An educational program on depressive disorders for general practitioners on Gotland: Background and evaluation. *Acta Psychiatrica Scandinavica, 79,* 19–26. http://doi.org/10.1111/j.1600-0447.1989.tb09229.x

Sabo, A. N., & Rand, B. (2000). The relational aspects of psychopharmacology. In A. N. Sabo & L. Havens (Eds.), *The real world guide to psychotherapy practice* (pp. 34–59). Cambridge, MA: Harvard University Press.

Saltzman, C., Luctgert, M. J., Roth, C. H., Creaser, J., & Howard, L. (1976). Formation of a therapeutic relationship: Experiences during the initial phase of psychotherapy as predictors of treatment duration and outcome. *Journal of Consulting and Clinical Psychology, 44,* 546–555. http://doi.org/10.1037/0022-006X.44.4.546

Sarbin, T. R. (1986). *Narrative psychology: The storied nature of human conduct.* New York, NY: Praeger.

Schauer, M., Neuner, F., & Elbert, T. (2012). *Narrative exposure therapy: A short-term treatment for traumatic stress disorders (2nd ed.).* Cambridge, MA: Hogrefe.

Schechter, M., & Goldblatt, M. (2011). Validation, empathy, and genuine relatedness. In K. Michel & D. A. Jobes (Eds.), *Building a therapeutic alliance with the suicidal patient* (pp. 93–107). Washington, DC: American Psychological Association.

Schmidtke, A., Bille-Brahe, U., DeLeo, D., Kerkhof, A., Bjerke, T., Crepet, P., . . . Sampaio-Faria, J. G. (1996). Attempted suicide in Europe: Rates, trends and sociodemographic characteristics of suicide attempters during the period 1989–1992. Results of the WHO/EURO Multicentre Study on Parasuicide. *Acta Psychiatrica Scandinavica, 93,* 327–338. http://doi.org/10.1111/j.1600-0447.1996.tb10656.x

Schmidtke, A., & Häfner, H. (1986). Die Vermittlung von Selbstmordmotivation und Selbstmordhandlung durch fiktive Modelle. Die Folgen der Fernsehserie "Tod eines Schülers" [The transmission of suicidal motivation and suicidal action through fiction modelling. Effect of the TV series "Death of a Student"]. *Nervenarzt, 57,* 502–510.

Schmidtke, A., & Schaller, S. (2000). The role of mass media in suicide prevention. In R. O'Connor, S. Platt, & J. Gordon (Eds.), *The international handbook of suicide and attempted suicide, policy and practice* (pp. 675–697). Chichester, UK: Wiley.

Schmidtke, A., Sell, R., Wohner, J., Löhr, C., & Tatsek, K. (2005). Epidemiologie von Suizid und Suizidversuch in Deutschland [Epidemiology of suicide and attempted suicide in Germany]. *Suizidprophylaxe, 32,* 87–99.

Shneidman, E. (1987). A psychological approach to suicide. In G. VandenBos & B. Bryant (Eds.), *Cataclysms, crises and catastrophies: Psychology in action.* Washington, DC: American Psychological Association.

Shneidman, E. S. (1985). *The definition of suicide: An essay.* New York, NY: Wiley.

Shneidman, E. S. (1993). Commentary: Suicide as psychache. *The Journal of Nervous and Mental Disease, 181,* 145–147. http://doi.org/10.1097/00005053-199303000-00001

Silverman, M. M., Berman, A. L., Sanddal, N. D., O'Carroll, P. W., & Joiner, T. E. (2007). Rebuilding the tower of babel: A revised nomenclature for the study of suicide and suicidal behaviors: Part 1: Background, rationale, and methodology. *Suicide and Life-Threatening Behavior, 37,* 248–263. http://doi.org/10.1521/suli.2007.37.3.264

Sinclair, J., & Green, J. (2005). Understanding resolution of deliberate self harm: Qualitative interview study of patients' experiences. *BMJ, 330,* 1112. http://doi.org/10.1136/bmj.38441.503333.8F

Skegg, K. (2005). Self-harm. *Lancet, 366,* 1471–1483. http://doi.org/10.1016/S0140-6736(05)67600-3

Slee, N., Garnefski, N., van der Leeden, R., Arensman, E., & Spinhoven, P. (2008). Cognitive-behavioural intervention for self-harm: Randomised controlled trial. *British Journal of Psychiatry, 192,* 202–211. http://doi.org/10.1192/bjp.bp.107.037564

Soloff, P. H., Fabio, A., Kelly, T. M., Malone, K. M., & Mann, J. J. (2005). High-lethality status in patients with borderline personality disorder. *Journal of Personality Disordprders, 19*, 386–399. http://doi.org/10.1521/pedi.2005.19.4.386

Sonneck, G., Etzersdorfer, E., & Nagel-Kuess, S. (1994). Imitative suicide on the Viennese subway. *Social Science & Medicine, 38*, 453–457. http://doi.org/10.1016/0277-9536(94)90447-2

Stack, S. (1983). The effect of religious commitment on suicide: A cross-national analysis. *Journal of Health and Social Behavior, 24*, 362–374. http://doi.org/10.2307/2136402

Stanley, B., & Brown, G. K. (2012). Safety planning intervention: A brief intervention to mitigate suicide risk. *Cognitive and Behavioral Practice, 19*, 256–264. http://doi.org/10.1016/j.cbpra.2011.01.001

Stanovich, K. E., & West, R. F. (2000). Individual differences in reasoning: Implications for the rationality debate? *Behavioral and Brain Sciences, 23*, 645–665. http://doi.org/10.1017/S0140525X00003435

Stenager, E. N., & Stenager, E. (2000). Physical illness and suicidal behavior. In v. H. K. Hawton K. (Ed.), *The international handbook of suicide and attempted suicide* (pp. 405–420). Chichester, UK: Wiley.

Stengel, E. (1964). *Suicide and attempted suicide.* Baltimore, MD: Penguin Books.

Substance Abuse and Mental Health Services Administration, Mental Health Services Administration. (2012). *Results from the 2011 national survey on drug use and health: Summary of national findings.* Rockville, MD: Author.

Suokas, J., Suominen, K., Isometsä, E., Ostamo, A., & Lönnqvist, J. (2001). Long-term risk factors for suicide mortality after attempted suicide: Findings of a 14-year follow-up study. *Acta Psychiatrica Scandinavica, 104*, 117–121. http://doi.org/10.1034/j.1600-0447.2001.00243.x

Suominen, K. H., Isometsä, E. T., Henriksson, M. M., Ostamo, A. I., & Lönnqvist, J. K. (1998). Inadequate treatment for major depression both before and after attempted suicide. *American Journal of Psychiatry, 155*, 1778–1780. http://doi.org/10.1176/ajp.155.12.1778

Suominen, K., Isometsä, E., Suokas, J., Haukka, J., Achte, K., & Lönnqvist, J. (2004). Completed suicide after a suicide attempt: A 37-year follow-up study. *American Journal of Psychiatry, 161*, 562–563. http://doi.org/10.1176/appi.ajp.161.3.562

Teicher, M. H., Glod, C., & Cole, J. O. (1990). Emergence of intense suicidal preoccupation during fluoxetine treatment. *American Journal of Psychiatry, 147*, 207–210. http://doi.org/10.1176/ajp.147.2.207

ten Have, M., de Graaf, R., Van Dorsselaer, S., Verdurmen, J., van't Land, H., Vollebergh, W., & Beekman, A. (2009). Incidence and course of suicidal ideation and suicide attempts in the general population. Canadian Journal of Psychiatry. *Revue Canadienne de Psychiatrie, 54*, 824–833.

Treolar, A. J., & Pinfold, T. J. (1993). Deliberate self-harm: An assessment of patients' attitudes to the care they receive. *Crisis, 14*, 83–89.

Valach, L., Michel, K., Dey, P., & Young, R. A. (2002). Self-confrontation interview with suicide attempters. *Counseling Psychology Quarterly, 15*, 1–22. http://doi.org/10.1080/09515070110101487

Valach, L., Michel, K., Young, R. A., & Dey, P. (2002). Attempted suicide stories: Suicide career, suicide project and suicide action. In L. Valach, R. A. Young, & M. J. Lynam (Eds.), *Action theory primer for applied research in the social sciences* (pp. 153–171). Westport, CT: Praeger.

Valach, L., Michel, K., Young, R. A., & Dey, P. (2006). Suicide attempts as social goal-directed systems of joint careers, projects, and actions. *Suicide and Life-Threatening Behavior, 36*, 651–660. http://doi.org/10.1521/suli.2006.36.6.651

Valach, L., Young, R. A., & Lynam, M. J. (2002). *Action theory: A primer for applied research in the social sciences.* Westport, CT: Praeger.

Valach, L., Young, R. A., & Michel, K. (2011). Understanding suicide as an action. In K. Michel & D. A. Jobes (Eds.), *Building a therapeutic alliance with the suicidal patient* (pp. 129–148). Washington, DC: American Psychological Association.

Van Heeringen, C., Jannes, S., Buylaert, W., Henderick, H., De Bacquer, D., & Van Remoortel, J. (1995). The management of non-compliance with referral to out-patient after-care among attempted suicide patients: A controlled intervention study. *Psychological Medicine, 25*, 963–970. http://doi.org/10.1017/S0033291700037454

Van Heeringen, C., & Marusic, A. (2003). Understanding the suicidal brain. *British Journal of Psychiatry, 183*, 282–284. http://doi.org/10.1192/bjp.183.4.282

Ventrice, D., Valach, L., Reisch, T., & Michel, K. (2010). Suicide attempters' memory traces of exposure to suicidal behavior: A qualitative pilot study. *Crisis, 31*, 93–99. http://doi.org/10.1027/0227-5910/a000013

Wadsworth, T., & Kubrin, C. E. (2007). Hispanic suicide in US metropolitan areas: Examining the effects of immigration, assimilation, affluence, and disadvantage. *American Journal of Sociology, 112,* 1848–1885.

Weinberg, I., Ronningstam, E., Goldblatt, M. J., & Maltsberger, J. T. (2011). Vicissitudes of the therapeutic alliance with suicidal patients: A psychoanalytic perspective. In K. Michel & D. A. Jobes (Eds.), *Building a therapeutic alliance with the suicidal patient* (pp. 293–316). Washington, DC: American Psychological Association APA Books.

Welu, T. C. (1977). A follow-up program for suicide attempters: Evaluation of effectiveness. *Suicide and Life-Threatening Behavior, 7,* 17–30.

Wenzel, A., Brown, G. K., & Beck, A. T. (2009). *Cognitive therapy for suicidal patients: Scientific and clinical applications.* Washington, DC: American Psychological Association. http://doi.org/10.1037/11862-000

Williams, J. M. G., & Pollock, L. R. (2000). The psychology of suicidal behaviour. In K. Hawton & K. van Heeringen (Eds.), *The international handbook of suicide and attempted suicide* (pp. 79–93). Chichester, UK: Wiley.

Williams, J. M. G., & Pollock, L. R. (2001). Psychological aspects of the suicidal process. In K. van Heeringen (Ed.), *Understanding suicidal behaviour: The suicidal process approach to research, treatment and prevention* (pp. 76–93). Chichester, UK: Wiley.

Williams, J. M. G., & Swales, M. (2004). The use of mindfulness-based approaches for suicidal patients. *Archives of Suicide Research, 8,* 315–329. http://doi.org/10.1080/13811110490476671

Williams, J. M., Mathews, A., & MacLeod, C. (1996). The emotional Stroop task and psychopathology. *Psychological Bulletin, 120,* 3–24. http://doi.org/10.1037/0033-2909.120.1.3

Williams, J. M., Teasdale, J. D., Segal, Z. V., & Soulsby, J. (2000). Mindfulness-based cognitive therapy reduces overgeneral autobiographical memory in formerly depressed patients. *Journal of Abnormal Psychology, 109,* 150–155. http://doi.org/10.1037/0021-843X.109.1.150

Wolfersdorf, M. (2000). *Der suizidale Patient in Klinik und Praxis: Suizidalität und Suizidprävention* [The suicidal patient in clinical care and practice: Suicidality and suicide prevention]. Stuttgart: Wissenschaftliche Verlagsgesellschaft.

Wolfersdorf, M. (2008). Suizidalität [Suicidality]. *Der Nervenarzt, 79,* 1319–1334. http://doi.org/10.1007/s00115-008-2478-2

Wolk-Wasserman, D. (1987). Contacts of suicidal neurotic and prepsychotic/psychotic patients and their significant others with public care institutions before the suicide attempt. *Acta Psychiatrica Scandinavica, 75,* 358–372. http://doi.org/10.1111/j.1600-0447.1987.tb02803.x

WHO Regional Office for Europe (1986). *Working group on prevention practices in suicide and attempted suicide.* Copenhagen, Denmark: Author.

World Health Organization. (2003). *Suicide prevention in Europe: The WHO European monitoring survey on national suicide prevention programs and strategies.* Copenhagen: WHO Regional Office for Europe.

World Health Organization. (2011a). *Figures and facts about suicide.* Geneva, Switzerland. Retrieved from http://www.who.int/menatl_health/prevention/suicide/country_reports/en/

World Health Organization. (2011b). *The international classification of diseases* (10th revision). Geneva, Switzerland: Author.

World Health Organization. (2013). *WHO mental health action plan 2013–2020.* Retrieved from http://www.who.int/mental_health/publications/action_plan/en/

World Health Organization. (2014a). *Suicide* (Fact sheet no. 398). Retrieved from http://www.who.int/mediacentre/factsheets/fs398/en/

World Health Organization. (2014b). *Preventing suicide: A global imperative.* Geneva, Switzerland: Author.

Yerevanian, B. I., Feusner, J. D., Koek, R. J., & Mintz, J. (2004). The dexamethasone suppression test as a predictor of suicidal behavior in unipolar depression. *Journal of Affecivet Disorders, 83,* 103–108. http://doi.org/10.1016/j.jad.2004.08.009

Young, R. A., Valach, L., Dillabough, J.-A., Dover, C., & Matthes, G. (1994). Career research from an action perspective: The self-confrontation procedure. *Career Development Quarterly, 43,* 185–196. http://doi.org/10.1002/j.2161-0045.1994.tb00857.x

Appendices

Appendix 1. Template Information Sheet for Patients

<<Letterhead>>

Brief Therapy After a Suicidal Crisis:
ASSIP (Attempted Suicide Short Intervention Program)

Dear Patient,

This brief four-session therapy followed by contact through regular letters is recommended as a routine procedure to patients who have attempted suicide. After attempted suicide, the risk of further suicidal crises is considerably increased for many years to come. Therefore, it is essential that with your help, we try to understand the background of your suicidal crisis, and that we develop safety strategies for the future. ASSIP brief therapy does not replace any other recommended follow-up treatment. However, we will make sure that, with your consent, health professionals involved in your treatment will be informed about the safety measures developed in ASSIP.

In the next few days you will be contacted by one of the persons who have signed below. If you are currently in an inpatient unit, we will first contact the doctor in charge of your treatment.

<<Therapist's name>>

Please detach

- -

I agree that a therapist of the ASSIP team can contact me regarding the brief therapy described above.

Last name: . . . . First name: . . . .

Date of birth: . . . .

Responsible health professional: . . . .

Probable further treatment: . . . .

I can be reached *by telephone*. Number: . . . .

Preferably from . . . . to . . . .

Please contact me *in writing*

Address: . . . .

or e-mail: . . . .

Date: . . . . Signature: . . . .

From: K. Michel & A. Gysin-Maillart: *ASSIP – Attempted Suicide Short Intervention Program*   © 2015 Hogrefe Publishing

Appendix 2. Template Information Sheet for Health Professionals

<<Letterhead>>

Brief Therapy After a Suicidal Crisis: ASSIP (Attempted Suicide Short Intervention Program)

This brief therapy is recommended as a routine procedure to all patients who have attempted suicide. A history of attempted suicide is the main risk factor for suicide and attempted suicide. The risk remains elevated for decades and is at its highest in the first year after a suicide attempt. ASSIP is a specific, structured therapy focusing on the patient's individual suicidality, aimed at a patient-oriented understanding of the background of the suicidal crisis, and at developing specific safety measures for the future. ASSIP does not replace any other recommended follow-up treatment, but therapists involved in the patient's treatment will be informed about the procedure and receive a copy of the written summary.

Patients who are admitted to the emergency department are routinely informed about ASSIP and asked to fill out the agreement form so that we can contact them in the psychiatric unit or at home.

Structure of ASSIP

This brief therapy consists of normally four sessions followed by subsequent contacts by letter.

- First session: Narrative interview focusing on the background of the suicidal crisis. The interview is video-recorded, with the patient's written consent.
- Second session: Video playback. Patient and therapist watch the recorded interview together, interrupting regularly for additional information. The patient receives a psycho-educational handout to read and comment on as a homework task.
- Third session: Completion of a written case formulation of the individual vulnerability and the typical triggering event(s) preceding a suicidal crisis. Individual preventive measures are developed in a collaborative manner, printed in a credit card size ("Hope Leporello") and handed to the patient.
- Fourth session (optional): Miniexposure. The safety strategies are practiced using the video-recorded narrative interview.
- Standardized letters. Contact with regular letters for 2 years; every 3 months in the first year, every 6 months in the second year.

Please send referrals with the separate patient's consent form to the ASSIP team. The patient will then be contacted.

<<Name, e-mail address, telephone number of the ASSIP team>>

Appendix 3. Homework Text: "Suicide Is Not a Rational Act"

Homework – ASSIP

Suicide Is Not a Rational Act

Many of us have moments in our lives in which we may consider suicide as a possible solution to a difficult life situation. This is quite normal. Many people would say that we have this freedom of choice. The state of mind of the acutely suicidal person, however, has little to do with freedom of choice.

Mental Pain

The acute suicidal crisis is usually the result of an experience that fundamentally threatens our sense of self. The associated state of mind is often described as intense psychological or mental pain. This pain may be worse than the most extreme physical pain. Often, it is triggered by a negative experience, such as a threatened or actual breakdown of a relationship, or by an experience of personal failure or loss of important personal goals. The situation becomes dangerous when we start to hate and reject ourselves because of self-blame – that is, when we start to turn against ourselves. When we see no solution to such a painful experience, a state of alarm will ensue, which may be difficult to control. Suicidal people report that they were not their usual self anymore and that they were acting in a trance-like state, that they felt disconnected from their physical body and felt no pain. These critical mental states are called *dissociation,* which means that the normal self-perception is disrupted. In such a condition it is practically impossible to think and act rationally. People lose faith that this experience of alarm and intense pain will ever subside.

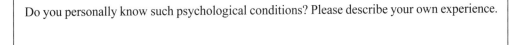

Do you personally know such psychological conditions? Please describe your own experience.

The Emotional Brain and the Rational Brain

Recent brain research has begun to shed some light on what happens in the brain in an acute suicidal crisis. Normally, our behavior is the result of the harmonious integration of two major brain regions: on the one hand, the emotional brain, basically located in the limbic system, and on the other, the rational brain, located in the frontal cortex (also referred to as the brain's CEO). The limbic system and, in particular, the amygdala are the brain areas responsible for the detection of threatening situations and for quick behavioral responses. Threatening situations trigger an acute stress response with a release of adrenaline into the blood. This is called a flight–fight reaction, a reaction pattern that can be found throughout evolution. Increased stress hormones (adrenaline and cortisol) drastically reduce the function of the frontal cortical areas, the part of the brain responsible for problem solving, planning, and rational thinking in accordance with our own biography. In a situation of acute emotional stress, these functions are no longer accessible.

From: K. Michel & A. Gysin-Maillart: ASSIP – Attempted Suicide Short Intervention Program   © 2015 Hogrefe Publishing

We would like to know if this makes sense to you. Can you please comment?

Acts of Self-Harm Will Be Stored in the Brain

Once we have experienced a suicidal crisis, particularly after a suicide attempt, such an out-of-the-ordinary emotionally stressful or even traumatic experience will be stored in the brain circuitry as a so-called *suicidal mode.* The suicidal mode is a brain condition learned and stored as a cognitive-emotional-behavioral state of mind, designed to deal with specific, extraordinary situations. This means that it will be reactivated again when triggered by a similar situation. Suicide as a solution will then be a readily available behavioral response to mental pain. It is therefore not surprising that attempted suicide is the main risk factor for later suicide or repeated suicide attempts. Unfortunately, the risk will be elevated for years. This is the reason it is so important to develop and establish effective safety strategies for future crises.

Your comments regarding your own past suicidal crises:

Factors Increasing Suicide Risk

Early traumatic experiences render an individual vulnerable to uncontrollable stress responses in emotionally threatening situations in adult life and therefore increase the risk of suicide. Such traumatic experiences include sexual abuse, maltreatment, violence in the family, but also emotional neglect and separation. They are typically experiences that in childhood and adolescence have already been associated with mental pain, and which left an enduring engram (memory trace). Because the frontal cortex matures up to early adulthood, the adolescent brain in particular is subject to impulsivity and aggression, both risk factors for suicide and attempted suicide.

Is it possible that early negative experiences could be a factor in your case?
Your comments:

Depression

Depression is an important risk factor for completed suicide. Depressed individuals tend to be ashamed and blame themselves for their condition. They lose hope that they will get better again. In a state of depression, it is difficult to seek help and talk about the loss of one's usual sense of self. Suicidal thoughts are frequent, and often not communicated.

In depression – which often is the result of emotionally stressful experiences – normal brain function is changed, and this pathological condition cannot be overcome by willpower. In particular, neural activity in the frontal cortex is reduced, problem-solving capacities are impaired, and self-perception tends to be negative ("I am a failure, I am a burden to my family, things will never get better"). All this may lead to the thought that suicide is the only solution. Therefore, it is extremely important to recognize depressive symptoms and to openly talk about suicidal thoughts. Mental health professionals know that depression can be successfully treated, and once people feel better, the suicidal impulses will disappear.

☐   I believe that depression is a factor in my case
☐   I may have other problems with mental health
Please describe:

You Should Know What to Do When You Are Suicidal

The way we deal with an emotional crisis differs individually and depends on a variety of factors. Many people can cope with mental pain, maybe because they have learned to trust that the seemingly unbearable condition will not last forever, but also maybe because their brain is better equipped to deal with extreme stress. However, for most people in times of crisis, it is important to turn to a person in whom they trust and to whom they can talk to about their inner turmoil. If a person has a history of attempted suicide, it is extremely important to be aware of early warning signs and to react before the suicidal mode is switched on, when emotional impulses and dissociation take over. After a suicide attempt it is extremely important to have a list of personal safety strategies, as a means to prevent the dangerous loss of reality. Such lists may include self-help strategies such as walking the dog or going to see a neighbor, but above all, they include names and contact information of persons one can turn to. These may be family members or friends, or it may be a crisis line number, emergency numbers of health professionals, such as a family doctor, psychiatrist, psychologist, etc., who will have the knowledge and experience to help a person to deal with an acute suicidal crisis.

In my case, I think the following strategies could be helpful:
1.
2.
3.
4.

Professionals and institutions I could turn to:
1.
2.
3.
4.

Please try to answer the questions, and take this handout to the next session.

Thank you!

<<Name, e-mail address, telephone number of ASSIP therapist>>

From: K. Michel & A. Gysin-Maillart: *ASSIP – Attempted Suicide Short Intervention Program*   © 2015 Hogrefe Publishing

Appendix 4. Assessment of Suicide Risk

When working with suicidal people, it is important that the therapist assesses the suicide risk and takes the according measures for the patient's protection. Because ASSIP has been developed as an add-on to treatment as usual, the authors in their work setting usually see patients that have been admitted to a psychiatric ward or are seen as outpatients as part of the usual clinical management after attempted suicide. Therefore, in this setting, the ASSIP therapist is not expected to do a full clinical assessment including psychiatric diagnosis and a thorough evaluation of suicide risk. If a patient is not under concurrent professional inpatient or outpatient care, it may be necessary to repeat the risk assessment by using the SSF at the end of each session. In case of acute suicide risk, admission to a secure psychiatric ward may be necessary.

Suicidal patients are often reluctant to talk about their suicidal intentions, particularly when bombarded with questions. Jobes (1995) has pointed out that, although a large number of suicide risk scales have been developed, very few of them are used in clinical practice. Scales for suicide risk assessment generally may provide an estimation of long-term suicide risk. The assessment of the current suicide risk (i.e., now and in the coming days) requires individual psychiatric exploration and assessment, ideally as a collaborative process, in connection with narrative exploration, an approach which Jobes called "therapeutic assessment." When seeing suicidal patients, we must bear in mind that they are often ashamed and have a low self-esteem. A basis for trust, allowing a realistic assessment of the current suicide risk, will only be possible when patients experience that they are taken seriously and that the therapist is trying to understand the personal context of their suicidal crisis. Jobes (2006, 2010) developed a semistructured interview model (Suicide Status Form [SSF-III], see Appendix 5), which in our experience is an excellent tool for the assessment of acute suicidality, consistent with the patient-oriented, collaborative approach used in ASSIP.

The authors use the SSF-III at the end of their first session, following the narrative interview. It is essential that the therapist and the patient sit side by side (see Figure 3 in Section 3.1.1) and that the therapist briefly explains the individual questions before patient fills out the form. It has proven useful to answer items 1 to 5 twice: first for the time of the recent suicide crisis, then again for the moment in the here and now. After the narrative interview, which is often emotionally charged, the SSF is a useful means of debriefing, due to its clearly structured set of questions focusing on common aspects of acute suicidality.

Studies on suicide risk factors (see also Section 2.2.3) have identified a large number of personal and clinical risk factors. Although they are relevant for the evaluation of long-term suicide risk, they are usually of little value in the assessment of acute suicidality. However, a comprehensive suicide risk assessment will, in addition to the SSF-III, include a list of questions related to relevant personal and clinical aspects of suicidality.

Distress, mental pain

What is the nature and level of the person's inner distress and pain?

What are the main sources of distress?

Meaning, motivation

What is the person's understanding of the actual predicament? How does the person see the meaning of recent events?

From: K. Michel & A. Gysin-Maillart: *ASSIP – Attempted Suicide Short Intervention Program*   © 2015 Hogrefe Publishing

What is motivating the person to harm himself or herself?

Does the person believe that it might be possible for their predicament to change and that they might be able to bring this about?

At-risk mental states

Mental states associated with increased suicide risk include hopelessness, despair, agitation, shame, anger, guilt, and psychotic symptoms. Clinicians should look for and directly inquire about such feelings. The psychiatric diagnosis of current depressive symptoms is considered to be a particular risk factor.

History of suicidal behavior

Has the person harmed himself or herself before?

What were the details and circumstances of the previous attempt/s?

Are there any similarities in the current circumstances?

Is there a history of suicide of a family member or friend?

Current suicidal thoughts

Are suicidal thoughts and feelings present?

What are these thoughts (determine the content – for example, guilt, delusions, or thoughts of reunion)?

When did these thoughts begin?

How frequent are they?

How persistent are they?

Can the person control them?

What has stopped the person from acting on these thoughts so far?

Circumstances of suicide attempt

Events that triggered the suicide attempt (relationship loss, job loss, other experiences of loss)

Has the person finalized personal business – for example, made a will, made arrangements for pets, debts, goodbyes, and giving away possessions?

Lethality of means

Is the chosen method irreversible – for example, shooting, jumping?

Has the person made a special effort to find out information about methods of suicide or do they have particular knowledge of lethal means?

Coping potential or capacity

Does the person have the capacity to enter into a therapeutic alliance/partnership?

Does the person recognize any personal strengths or effective coping strategies?

Adapted from NSW Department of Health. (2004). *Framework for Suicide Risk Assessment and Management for NSW Health Staff*. Sydney, Australia: Author.

How has the person managed previous life events and stressors? What are possible problem-solving strategies?

Are there any social or community supports (e.g., family, friends, church, general practitioner)? Can the person use these?

Is the person motivated to comply with the treatment plan?

Does the person have a history of aggression or impulsive behavior? (Aggression and impulsivity make risk status less predictable.)

Management of suicide risk

Steps to be taken after attempted suicide should be directly related to the assessment of a patient's suicidality. An important aspect is the therapist's assessment confidence. Refusal of help, little rapport, ambivalence, and poor engagement in the assessment are reasons to decide on high suicide risk. Other high-risk factors are severe depression, psychotic symptoms, substance intoxication, anger, and hostility. For patients at high risk or where there is a low assessment confidence in the risk level assessed, or high changeability in the person or their environment, a face-to-face reassessment should occur within 24 hr. Contingency planning for rapid reassessment should be implemented.

The decision to hospitalize a patient should be made on clinical grounds and, if possible, with the involvement of the patient.

High-risk patients need a secure inpatient environment, with or without involuntary commitment. Close monitoring should be provided. Risk assessment should be repeated within 24 hr. Special antisuicidal measures, such as removing dangerous objects, rules for going out, limited contact with others, may be necessary.

Medium or low risk patients may be followed up with an outpatient appointment, ideally within 48 hr and, if possible, with the health professional who carried out the initial clinical assessment. Patients missing their appointments should be contacted by telephone or through a home visit.

The use of psychotropic medication depends on the diagnosis and severity of psychopathology. In the case of acute suicidality, benzodiazepines may be helpful to reduce tension.

Reliance on so-called no-suicide contracts is not recommended. Research has shown that such contracts were in place for most of the suicides that occurred in an inpatient, acute care facility (Busch, Fawcett, & Jacobs, 2003; Kroll, 2000). As a practice alternative to a no-suicide contract, Rudd et al. (2006) recommend a commitment-to-treatment statement, which aims at securing treatment engagement.

Recommended Literature

NSW Department of Health. (2004). *Framework for suicide risk assessment and management for NSW health staff, 2004.* Sydney, Australia: Author. Retrieved from http://www.health.nsw.gov.au/mhdao/programs/mh/Publications/framework-suicide-risk-assess.pdf

American Psychiatric Association. (2003). *Practice guideline for the assessment and treatment of patients with suicidal behaviors.* Retrieved from http://psychiatryonline.org/pb/assets/raw/sitewide/practice_guidelines/guidelines/suicide.pdf

Appendix 5. Suicide Status Form (SSF-III)

For details of how to administer this form, see Section 3.4.3 and the Box "Suicide Status Form (SSF-III)."

Section A (Patient):	
Rank	Rate and fill out each item according to how you feel right now Then rank in order of importance 1 to 5 (1 = *most important* to 5 = *least important*).
	1) RATE PSYCHOLOGICAL PAIN (*hurt, anguish, or misery in your mind, **not** stress, **not** physical pain*): **Low pain: 1 2 3 4 5 :High pain** What I find most painful is:
	2) RATE STRESS (*your general feeling of being pressured or overwhelmed*): **Low stress: 1 2 3 4 5 :High stress** What I find most stressful is:
	3) RATE AGITATION (*emotional urgency; feeling that you need to take action; **not** irritation; **not** annoyance*): **Low agitation: 1 2 3 4 5 :High agitation** I most need to take action when:
	4) RATE HOPELESSNESS (*your expectation that things will not get better no matter what you do*): **Low hopelessness: 1 2 3 4 5 :High hopelessness** I am most hopeless about:
	5) RATE SELF-HATE (*your general feeling of disliking yourself; having no self-esteem; having no self-respect*): **Low self-hate: 1 2 3 4 5 :High self-hate** What I hate most about myself is:
N/A	6) RATE OVERALL RISK OF SUICIDE: **Extremely low risk: 1 2 3 4 5 :Extremely high risk** **(will not kill self) (will kill self)**

1. How much is being suicidal related to thoughts and feelings about <u>yourself</u>?   **Not at all: 1 2 3 4 5 : completely**
2. How much is being suicidal related to thoughts and feelings about <u>others</u>?   **Not at all: 1 2 3 4 5 : completely**

Please list your reasons for wanting to live and your reasons for wanting to die. Then rank in order of importance 1 to 5.

Rank	REASONS FOR LIVING	Rank	REASONS FOR DYING

I wish to live to the following extent:	Not at all: 0 1 2 3 4 5 6 7 8 : Very much
I wish to die to the following extent:	Not at all: 0 1 2 3 4 5 6 7 8 : Very much

The one thing that would help me no longer feel suicidal would be:

Appendix 6. Consent Form For Video Recording

<<Letterhead>>

Brief Therapy After a Suicidal Crisis:
ASSIP (Attempted Suicide Short Intervention Program)

Video Recording of the Initial Interview

Consent Form

The undersigned gives consent for the video recording of the therapy session.

The recording will used in the second session (video playback) and in the fourth session (rehearsal of safety strategies). In addition, the video recording may be used exclusively by the responsible ASSIP therapist and his or her supervisor.

The recording, including the person's name and data as well as the names and information regarding all other persons mentioned in the interview, will be strictly protected against any unauthorized access. The ASSIP therapist confirms with the signature below their responsibility for the confidentiality agreement.

The undersigned patient has the right to revoke this agreement at any time and to request the deletion of the video recording.

Date:. . . . .

I confirm that I have been informed about the purpose of the video recording and that I have read and understood the content of this agreement.

Patient signature: . . . .

I confirm that I am responsible for the maintenance of confidentiality as stated above.

Therapist signature: . . . .

From: K. Michel & A. Gysin-Maillart: *ASSIP – Attempted Suicide Short Intervention Program*   © 2015 Hogrefe Publishing

Appendix 7. Case Examples 1 and 2 With Sample Letters and Leporellos

Case Example 1: Ms. M.

<<Letterhead>>

Brief Therapy After a Suicidal Crisis: ASSIP (Attempted Suicide Short Intervention Program)

Ms. M., Sessions April 14, May 2, and May 9, 2013

Dear Ms. M.,

As discussed, here is my attempt to summarize the main points from our conversations on the background of your suicidal crisis. The following text is written in the first person, as it is your story.

1. Background

I had a difficult childhood and also later in life had many negative experiences. I was an unwanted fourth child and fell ill with meningitis in my childhood. During the day we were in the care of a child minder who was not interested in us. At school I became chubby and was often teased. My father beat me often, and then I had to start an apprenticeship that did not suit me. Throughout my life I have always tried to make something of myself. I took further training and opened my own workshop and gave courses. The boss treated me badly in the firm where I had worked for a long time, and for the first time I was prescribed medication. I left and started working in fashion sales, but here too, I experienced power struggles, and above all a lot of pressure from my superiors, which led to my first breakdown. I then started having problems with my health, in particular with my weight and numerous operations.

I married early at the age of 19, and I have two children who were both planned and wanted. After 23 years of marriage I got divorced. My first suicide attempt was connected to my ex-husband's new girlfriend who made a derogatory remark about my figure when I first went to visit them. It made me feel so ugly and completely worthless, and I wanted to put an end to my life.

Since then I've been treated for depression again and again and have been in the psychiatric hospital six times, usually following a suicide attempt. Recently I had more negative experiences: after a visit to the dentist, my cheek was swollen for days, my mother was picking at me, but above all my ex-husband forgot my birthday for the first time in 40 years. Ten days ago, when I was filling up my medication box, I suddenly had the impulsive thought "Life is crap, there's no point anymore, I can't fight anymore." My boyfriend was out of the house for a short time, and automatically, without thinking, I swallowed all the medication that I had got ready for the week. I can't actually say how it happened. My boyfriend called the ambulance, and I was taken to the emergency department and from there back to the psychiatric hospital.

We have seen that you had a difficult start in life, and throughout life you have often managed to overcome adverse experiences, but that there were again and again situations where your self-esteem collapsed. These are dangerous situations where as a sudden impulse suicide appears as a solution to extreme pain. We have seen that in order to prevent you from getting into the same – dangerous – situation again, it is important to take precautionary measures.

From: K. Michel & A. Gysin-Maillart: *ASSIP – Attempted Suicide Short Intervention Program*   © 2015 Hogrefe Publishing

2. The following measures are important for my safety in the future:

Helpful long-term measures:

- Regular therapy with Dr. S. and appointments with my GP, Dr. K.
- Medication is important to prevent relapse of depression.
- My partner should be in charge of medication
- Telling people in whom I trust what bothers me (partner, Dr. S., daughter)

Warning signs:

- When my feelings suddenly change
- Feeling of tightness in the chest, I can't get enough air
- Mood: Sadness, despair
- Thoughts: "I'm worthless," "life is pointless"
- Impulse to take an overdose

Safety strategies against suicide:

First

1. Pause for a moment and consider my thoughts and feelings
2. Get some fresh air
3. Take a bath ("winding down")
4. Talk to my daughter (Tel. no. ....)
5. Lorazepam to reduce tension

Acute

Call somebody!

6. Dr. S.............,   Tel. no. . . . .
7. Partner A.......,   Tel. no. . . . .
8. Prof. M..........,   Tel. no. . . . .
9. Duty doctor in outpatients clinic (24 hr!), Tel. no. . . . .
10. Emergency department,   Tel. no. . . . .

Established together on May 9, 2013

Approved:

Ms. M.   Prof. K. M.

. . . .
Signature   Signature

Copies: Dr. S., Dr. K.

From: K. Michel & A. Gysin-Maillart: *ASSIP – Attempted Suicide Short Intervention Program*   © 2015 Hogrefe Publishing

Hope Leporello for Ms. M.

Helpful long-term measures:
- Regular therapy with Dr. S. and appointments with GP, Dr. K.
- Medication is important to prevent relapse of depression.
- Partner should be in charge of medication
- Telling people in whom I trust what bothers me (partner, Dr. S., daughter)

Warning signs:
- When my feelings suddenly change
- Feeling of tightness in the chest, I can't get enough air
- Mood: Sadness, despair
- Thoughts: "I'm worthless, life is pointless"
- Impulse to take an overdose

Safety strategies against suicide:
First
1. Pause for a moment and consider my thoughts and feelings
2. Get some fresh air
3. Take a bath ("winding down")
4. Talk to my daughter (Tel. no. ....)
5. Lorazepam to reduce tension

Acute
Call somebody!
6. Dr. S.   Tel. no. . . . .
7. Partner A.   Tel. no. . . . .
8. Prof. M.   Tel. no. . . . .
9. Duty doctor in outpatients (24 hr!),
                            Tel. no. . . . .
10. Emergency department, Tel. no. . . . .

From: K. Michel & A. Gysin-Maillart: *ASSIP – Attempted Suicide Short Intervention Program*   © 2015 Hogrefe Publishing

Case Example 2: Mr. K.

<<Letterhead>>

Brief Therapy After a Suicidal Crisis:
ASSIP (Attempted Suicide Short Intervention Program)

Mr. K.

Sessions January 3, January 10, and January 17, 2013

Dear Mr. K.,

As discussed, here is my attempt at summarizing the main points from our conversations on the background of your suicidal crisis. The following text is written in the first person, as it is your story.

1. Background

My story starts in early childhood. As a small boy I was beaten by my father. He was out of work and drank a lot. I learnt very early on to be careful and to keep my feelings to myself. The feeling of inadequacy was very strong in me because whatever I did, no matter how much I tried to defend myself, there was no point, I couldn't protect myself and was alone and helpless.

These negative experiences had an effect on my character. The school alerted the authorities, and I was put in a home. I soon realized that I was still alone, and that I'd have to look for myself. I couldn't rely on anyone, I felt abandoned.

Very early on, I felt the wish to die, I couldn't see any way out. For years I tried to build my own life, not to think about it anymore or to talk about it and to be strong. But I suffered again and again from nightmares, was afraid of close relationships and felt like a failure.

About a year ago I started a new job in a company I liked. At the beginning I felt that I had finally found the right place. But then the reorganization started, and I got a new superior. He put more pressure on me each day, criticized me continually, wanted me to do overtime without pay. No matter what I did, it was never good enough. I felt blocked, a loser, couldn't sleep properly any more, withdrew from the people around me. At the same time, the problems in my relationship increased, I wasn't ready to make the next step (moving in together), then my girlfriend left me 2 months ago. She was fed up with waiting for me. When my uncle told me that I had time until the end of the year to repay the loan for my studies, it all became too much for me. How could I tell the only person who had always been there for me, that I wouldn't be able to do it?

I couldn't see any other solution than ending my life. So, 1 month ahead, I planned to kill myself with my gun. I started lying to people, stopped paying my bills. I shut myself up at home and didn't go out. On that day I got a bottle of whisky ready and drank half the bottle. When I opened the ammunition box, I knew that there was no way back. But then the phone rang, it was my uncle, and he could tell that something was wrong with me. He came to my house and took me to the emergency department where I received help".

In our talks together, we saw very clearly that there is an important issue that is anchored in your very early childhood. You had to take responsibility for your own life, engaging yourself in work. Pressure and rejection deeply hurt you, and the old impulse of giving up emerged again. Losing the one person you trusted triggered thoughts such as "There's no point, you can't do anything about it."

From: K. Michel & A. Gysin-Maillart: *ASSIP – Attempted Suicide Short Intervention Program*   © 2015 Hogrefe Publishing

2. The following measures are important for my safety in the future:

Helpful long-term measures:

- Find a therapist for long-term psychotherapy
- Learn to accept myself ("I'm ok the way I am!").
- Tackle problems step by step: learn to cope with stress
- Learn to get help when things become too much

Warning signs:

- Thinking in circles ("I'm wrong," "it's my fault")
- Intense feeling of being overwhelmed
- Helplessness, anger
- Problems sleeping
- Shutting myself up at home
- Not keeping important appointments, not opening the mail!

Safety strategies against suicide:

First

1. Physical activity: do sports
2. Read an thrilling book
3. Reduce tension – for example, play a computer game

Acute

Contact a health professional:

4. Psychiatrist, Dr. A. (Tel. no. ....)
5. ASSIP therapist (Tel. no ....), if necessary leave a message
6. Contact crisis team of outpatient dept. (Tel. no. ....)
7. Go to the emergency department of the general hospital

Developed together on January 17, 2013

Approved:

Mr. K.   A. G.-M

. . . .

Signature   Signature

Copies: Dr. A., Crisis Team

Hope Leporello for Mr. K.

Helpful long-term measures:
- Find a therapist for long-term therapy
- Learn to accept myself ("I'm ok the way I am!")
- Tackle problems step by step: learn to cope with stress
- Learn to get help when things become too much

Warning signs:
- Thinking in circles ("I'm wrong, it's my fault")
- Intense feeling of being overwhelmed
- Helplessness, anger
- Problems sleeping
- Shutting myself up at home
- Not keeping important appointments, not opening the mail!

Safety strategies against suicide:
First
8. Physical activity: do sports
9. Read an exciting book
10. Reduce tension, for example, play a computer game

Acute
Contact a professional:
11. Psychiatrist, Dr. A. (Tel. no. ....)
12. ASSIP therapist (Tel. no ....), if necessary leave a message
13. Contact crisis team of outpatient dept. (Tel. no. ....)
14. Go to the emergency department of the general hospital

From: K. Michel & A. Gysin-Maillart: *ASSIP – Attempted Suicide Short Intervention Program*   © 2015 Hogrefe Publishing

Appendix 8. Standardized Letters: First Letter (At 3 Months)

<<Letterhead>>

<<title>> <<first name>> <<last name>>
<<address line>>
<<address line>>

<<place, date>>

<<Dear Mr. ..., >>
<<Dear Ms. ...,>>

Three months have passed since your last appointment with me. I hope that things are going well for you. Let me remind you that if necessary you can contact us at any time. In case I am not available, please ask to be put through to our emergency team or emergency doctor (<<Tel. No.>>), they are available 24 hours.

Should things get difficult again for you, please remember the safety strategies we have developed. You must not let things get out of control so that suddenly you only see the one solution. Life is too valuable. As we believe that it can be life-saving for patients to know they can contact someone, you will receive a short note from us from time to time over a period of 2 years.

I would be pleased to hear from you if you would like to write a few lines, but you are not required to do so.

You will receive a next letter in 3 months' time. If you no longer wish to receive our letters, please let me know by phone or by e-mail.

Best wishes,

<<Therapist's name>>

<<E-mail address>>

From: K. Michel & A. Gysin-Maillart: *ASSIP – Attempted Suicide Short Intervention Program*   © 2015 Hogrefe Publishing

Appendix 9. Standardized Letters: Second Letter (At 6 Months)

<<Letterhead>>

<<title>> <<first name>> <<last name>>
<<address line>>
<<address line>>

<<place, date>>

<<Dear Mr. ..., >>
<<Dear Ms. ...,>>

Six months have passed since your last appointment with me. I hope you are well. You receive a few lines from us several times a year because we know that even a long time after a suicidal crisis, the danger is never completely gone.

Remember that even in a situation that appears at the time to be unbearable, you can pause for a few minutes, take an observer's look at your feelings, thoughts, and body sensations from a neutral position. Try to accept what you perceive ("At the moment that's just how it is. It is neither good nor bad"). Pain, mental pain, does not last forever. Suicidal impulses subside after a certain time. Wait until you feel that the level of agitation goes down.

Use your Hope Leporello we have developed together.

It often helps to talk to someone, to put things into perspective again. Don't forget that you can get in touch with us at any time. In case I am not available, please ask to be put through to our emergency team or emergency doctor (<<Tel. No.>>), they are available 24 hours.

I would be pleased to hear from you if you would like to write a few lines, but you are not required to do so.

You will receive a next letter in 3 months' time. If you no longer wish to receive our letters, please let me know by phone or by e-mail.

Best wishes,

<<Therapist's name>>

<<E-mail address>>

From: K. Michel & A. Gysin-Maillart: *ASSIP – Attempted Suicide Short Intervention Program*   © 2015 Hogrefe Publishing

Appendix 10. Standardized Letters: Third Letter (At 9 Months)

<<Letterhead>>

<<title>> <<first name>> <<last name>>
<<address line>>
<<address line>>

<<place, date>>

<<Dear Mr. ..., >>
<<Dear Ms. ...,>>

Nine months have passed since your last appointment with me. I hope that you are well. You receive a few lines from us several times a year because we know that even a long time after a suicidal crisis, the danger is never completely gone.

Experience has shown that even if things go well for a long period of time, something can suddenly happen to bring up suicidal thoughts again. If a person in the past has been close to attempting suicide or has attempted suicide, things will become dangerous again very quickly; the plan of suicide as a possible solution remains stored in the brain for years, and can all of a sudden be reactivated. I hope that your Hope Leporello is still in your pocket.

It is important to recognize *warning signs* early on. Withdrawing is always a bad solution. Talking to someone in times of crisis will help to change the perspective. That is why we would like to remind you with this letter that you can call us at any time. In case I am not available, please ask to be put through to our emergency team or emergency doctor (<<Tel. No.>>), they are available 24 hours.

I would be pleased to hear from you if you would like to write a few lines, but you are not required to do so.

You will receive a next letter in 3 months' time. If you no longer wish to receive our letters, please let me know by phone or by e-mail.

Best wishes,

<<Therapist's name>>

<<E-mail address>>

From: K. Michel & A. Gysin-Maillart: *ASSIP – Attempted Suicide Short Intervention Program*   © 2015 Hogrefe Publishing

Appendix 11. Standardized Letters: Fourth Letter (At 12 Months)

<<Letterhead>>

<<title>> <<first name>> <<last name>>
<<address line>>
<<address line>>

<<place, date>>

<<Dear Mr. ..., >>
<<Dear Ms. ...,>>

Another 3 months have passed since my last letter to you. I hope you are well. I am sure you understand why, for a certain period of time, we write letters to people who have come to us after a crisis: it is because we know that in the years following a suicide attempt the risk of another suicidal crises remains. It is important that you should know what to do in the event of another crisis. We believe that there is always another solution than suicide. Remember that however bad the mental pain is, it will always subside. Don't lose your head if things get critical again but instead:

- Pause for a few minutes, take an observer's look at your feelings, thoughts, and body sensations from a neutral position. Try to accept what you perceive. Wait until you feel that the level of agitation goes down;
- Use your personal Hope Leporello;
- Find someone to talk to – sometimes it even helps to talk about something quite mundane;
- Try to reach your family doctor or therapist;
- Call us; in case I am not available, please ask to be put through to our emergency team or emergency doctor (<<Tel. No.>>), they are available 24 hours;
- Go straight to the emergency department of the nearest hospital.

I would be pleased to hear from you if you would like to write a few lines, but you are not required to do so.

You will receive a next letter in 6 months' time. If you no longer wish to receive our letters, please let me know by phone or by e-mail.

Best wishes,

<<Therapist's name>>

<<E-mail address>>

From: K. Michel & A. Gysin-Maillart: *ASSIP – Attempted Suicide Short Intervention Program*   © 2015 Hogrefe Publishing

Appendix 12. Standardized Letters: Fifth Letter (At 18 Months)

<<Letterhead>>

<<title>> <<first name>> <<last name>>
<<address line>>
<<address line>>

<<place, date>>

<<Dear Mr. ..., >>
<<Dear Ms. ...,>>

Six months have passed since the last letter. I hope you are well. This is the last but one letter you will receive from us.

I would like to remind you again that a long-term emergency scenario is needed in the event of another crisis – although I hope of course that this never happens again to you. For this reason it is important to keep a list of emergency strategies in a place where you can easily find it again. Do you still carry your Hope Leporello with you? Pease don't forget that if things become difficult again that you shouldn't wait too long before seeking help – either from your family doctor or psychiatrist (your therapist) or from us.

If necessary call us; in case I am not available, please ask to be put through to our emergency team or emergency doctor (<<Tel. No.>>), they are available 24 hours.

I would be pleased to hear from you if you would like to write a few lines, but you are not required to do so.

Best wishes,

<<Therapist's name>>

<<E-mail address>>

Appendix 13. Standardized Letters: Sixth Letter (Last Letter)

<<Letterhead>>

<<title>> <<first name>> <<last name>>
<<address line>>
<<address line>>

<<place, date>>

<<Dear Mr. ..., >>
<<Dear Ms. ...,>>

This is the last letter you will receive from me. In these letters I tried to remind you that after a suicidal crisis a certain risk remains, and that it is important to know what to do in a crisis so that it doesn't become life-threatening. I hope, of course, that everything is going well and that you have not had any more critical moments, and that you won't have any in the future. Still, I recommend that you always carry your personal Hope Leporello with you.

As always, I would like to remind you that you can call us at any time. In case I am not available, please ask to be put through to our emergency team or emergency doctor (<<Tel. No. >>), they are available 24 hours. Or try to reach your family doctor or therapist. In an emergency you can go straight to the emergency department of the nearest hospital.

I would be pleased to receive from you – either in writing or by telephone – a brief feedback on how things have been going during the past 2 years. If I don't hear from you, then I wish you all the best for the future.

With best regards,

<<Therapist's name>>

<<E-mail address>>

From: K. Michel & A. Gysin-Maillart: *ASSIP – Attempted Suicide Short Intervention Program*   © 2015 Hogrefe Publishing

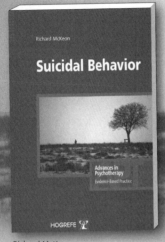
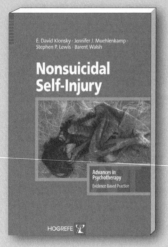
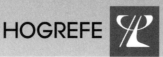

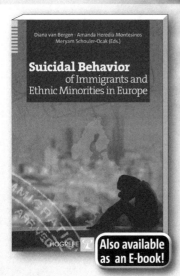
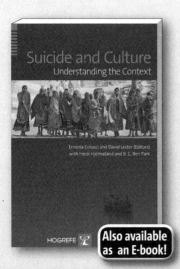
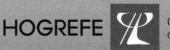

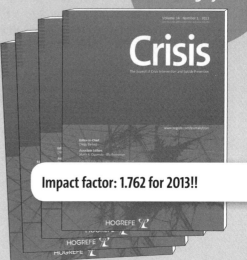 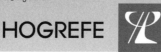